PRAISE FOR STEPHANIE HREHIRCHUK

What I find refreshing and intriguing is to read material that is so blatantly honest and revealing while providing a path to alternative self-discovery and self-help. I believe this can be one book that makes Energy Healing and Yoga practices more easily approachable for women who are not already familiar with these healing modalities.

— K.K., CALGARY, ALBERTA

Hrehirchuk's warm, relatable voice as narrator will keep readers invested, while leading them to accept that they too could aspire to such a spiritual journey. The witty chapter titles provide a humorous and playful reprieve from the more serious underlying subject matter—rehabilitating oneself physically and spiritually. Hrehirchuk powerfully emphasizes the connection between the physical and psychological. The detailed acknowledgment of the narrator's growth over her year of yoga is inspiring, funny, and heartwarming, and the narrative comes full circle at the end, focusing on the blessings of family.

— THE BOOKLIFE PRIZE

AN ACCIDENTAL AWAKENING

IT'S NOT ABOUT YOGA; IT'S ABOUT FAMILY

STEPHANIE HREHIRCHUK

Edited by
MARAYA LOZA KOXAHN

ANNA'S ANGELS PRESS

For my Family

Angie,
You were part
of this
journey:
this dream
realized.

With love!
Stephanie
A.

CONTENTS

PART VIII
CROWN CHAKRA

PROLOGUE

THE SPINE IS THE LADDER OF THE SOUL

~ The Trigger ~

Didn't I already get up this morning? I stared at the familiar black dress socks folded together in that balled-up way Mom had taught me to fold socks as a kid. The socks lay under the bed, bits of cat hair and dust bunnies clinging to them. *Wait. Under the bed? Why am I on the floor?* I shifted my gaze and saw Steve's panicked face hovering over me.

"You passed out in my arms," he said. "I had to set you on the floor." His expression shifted from fear to relief. "You were out cold... but your eyes were open the whole time. I thought about grabbing that pen, removing the ink cartridge and jabbing the shell MacGyver-style into your neck as a makeshift tracheotomy."

"Thank you for refraining," I managed. I couldn't tell if he was relieved or disappointed he didn't get the chance.

"Two flights of stairs. We can do it," Steve lifted me under the arms, enough to decompress the spine, but not so much as to strain the injury. I focused on my breath, resistant to waste energy on a response, and thankful for Steve's lean six-foot frame, constructed from years of hockey.

"You'll have to pick me up. I can't lift my leg."

Getting into the car forced me to seek reserves of strength hiding in my will and my bones. I found none. We needed to make it downtown to Aunt Joyce's treatment table for decompression. Luckily I had a chiropractor in my family. With the seat fully reclined, street lamps and overpass signs whizzed by as I peered over the dashboard on the seemingly endless drive downtown.

Days earlier I had woken with a stiff lower back. I assumed it would work itself out during the day as I headed downtown to meet with an early morning client. After work, I skipped Steve's and my regular ball hockey league and opted to hit the gym to work out my back. I woke the following morning more sore than ever.

The phone had rung and I'd raced downstairs to catch it before it went to voicemail. My foot slipped off the edge of the carpeted bottom step and I slammed down on my butt. A bolt of pain shot up my spine like a reverse lightning strike. I gingerly stood, took the last few steps to the kitchen and returned the missed call. By the end of the conversation, electricity radiated down the backs of my legs like the noisy neon sign at an all-night diner. I gripped the stair railing, a foreign feeling under my fingers, to help me back upstairs. Steve returned home after work to find me lying on the bed, still in my nightgown.

Aunt Joyce was my first call for help. She determined I had at least one herniated disc, likely torn, which kept me immobilized and forced me to leave my clients and my job as a personal trainer. With twenty years of athleticism, I was no stranger to injury and broken bones. The pain of those paled to what I endured while performing the simple movements I had once taken for granted. A mere sneeze would send me reeling. Even the excruciating collarbone break of 1999 had nothing on the spinal injury of 2003.

I relied upon Steve for meals, meds and to lift me out of bed and support my weight during the arduous, painful trips to the washroom. It was during one of the bathroom expeditions that I had passed out from the pain and ended up face-to-face with a pair of socks on the bedroom floor. The last thing I remembered was the jolt of electricity that fried my circuits. A sharp inhale caught in my throat. My body activated autopilot and shut down. Then the bedroom floor and a rush of fire through my torso as systems came back online. I was thirty-one years-old, less than two months from my wedding and unable to walk. Thirty-three days I lay in bed, pacified by pain.

Thanks to Steve's care, Aunt Joyce's prescription for natural remedies such as kava kava and valerian root, regular decompression sessions on her treatment table and my eventual surrender, I recovered enough to get back on my feet and resume training. As if I learned nothing from the experience, I returned to the gym and my trainer-brain that reconciled the recumbent bike as suitable cardio. My hands pressed firmly into the handles of the bike to support my upper body weight and take pressure off my lower discs. My legs pedaled away the lost time and fitness, in preparation for our beach wedding in Maui.

My pursuit of a beach body overshadowed the possibility of feeling grateful just to walk again. I continued to heal, eager to return to my previous self and unaware that option was no longer on the table. My soul had begun to climb the ladder of my spine: testing the strength of each rung for life ahead. It knew what was coming: marriage and children. I was in poor shape to support its weight.

~Same Me, Different Struggle~

ONE WEDDING, two small children, four years and one house later, I was a licensed Realtor with a personal training studio in my walkout basement, and my plate was full; my life was full. With snow thick on the ground and daylight at its shortest, I sat at the kitchen table with my cup of lemon tea, the kids eating breakfast and Steve off to work.

I spent more time in this room than any other: breakfast, lunch, dinner, snacks in between. I was grateful for my children, my husband and my home, but the fog in my head kept me from *feeling* gratitude. I thought about it but I don't believe I knew how it felt. I certainly couldn't describe the feeling of gratitude at the time. Maybe the fog was in my heart. In spite of understanding my good fortune of a loving family, a home, clients, friends and a great job, what I really wanted to know was: *is there life outside this kitchen?*

I wanted to scream it, as if someone would answer and lead me out of the room and the fog. I felt as though years had passed since I knew anything outside of these walls: my likes, dislikes, interests, desires, passions, goals, purpose, joy. I had lost myself in this kitchen.

In an attempt to improve my energy and outlook on life, I booked a reflexology session at a local wellness centre. Maybe some *me* time would lift my spirits. My face felt heavy. Frown lines etched the infamous elevens between my brows. No matter how much I massaged them, the grooves remained like tire tracks carved into once supple earth, now baked in place by years of heat.

My body felt heavy, exhausted from years of sleepless nights, days filled with motherly duties and my drive for professional success. Despite my physical activity and strength, I felt frail.

"Come, lie down and get comfortable." The reflexology therapist cooed. I melted into her treatment table and pulled up the fleece blanket. She pressed her thumbs into the soles of my feet. Tension poured from my body as I settled in for the hour-long treatment.

"I can't work on you in this state." She abruptly stood and moved to my head. "Would you mind if I did a bit of Reiki?"

I had no idea of Reiki. *Wait a minute, what state?* Feeling emotionally nourished in her care, I agreed. My eyes closed. I felt her hands flap and wave above me. My skin tingled, similar to when a hair stylist gives a great scalp massage during shampoo. The waving and tingling continued for five or ten minutes, then she returned to my feet.

When she finished the session, I couldn't pry myself from her table. I wanted to nap there for hours — how I felt much of the time during those days, as if sleep would consume me if I sat for a moment. My tired state was more than lack of sleep. Although I blamed it on the sleepless nights, the truth was I had pushed myself too hard for too long. Constantly expecting more and better from myself, I strove to be the top marketer, accomplished wife and perfect mother. I pushed my body even harder. I rarely declared myself satisfied with life — well, my performance in life — and seldom gave myself permission to just be. The last time I allowed myself to relax, completely stop and relax, was when my spinal injury had demanded it.

I returned home from the appointment and stood in the kitchen, looking out at the mountains as I did every day at sunset, as if somewhere out there lived the real me. That day the sunset looked different. I glimpsed a moment in that sunset. I *felt* a moment ... a spark of joy, a lightness of being.

The sky looked bluer and the sun shone brighter. The mountains stood intimately closer. I felt lighter.

I remember getting a new pair of prescription glasses at nineteen and putting them on for the first time to look at the night sky. The stars were no longer fuzzy dots against a dark canvas. They were pinpoints of light: clear and sharp. I took off my glasses and put them on again several times to compare the two perspectives. I remember thinking, Wow, is this how everyone else sees the world?

I knew in that moment, standing in my kitchen and staring out at those mountains, that *this* was the way life was meant to be seen. Like Dorothy had stepped out of black and white and emerged in Technicolor to skip on the path of gold, I too saw it before me. In that moment, I became aware of my fog and the nature of its illusion. It lasted only a moment but the awareness carved itself in my mind.

I booked two hours with the same practitioner at the wellness center for the following weekend. One hour of reflexology to satisfy my rational side — since I failed to comprehend how she could have flapped away my fog — and one hour of Reiki, because if that dispersed the haze, sign me up for life.

After that session, I dropped reflexology and returned several times for Reiki alone. The treatments began to restore my energy, not the kind received from food, more like life force energy. I no longer dragged my face around the house. Laughter returned and extended my short fuse. After years of helping clients with weight loss for the body, I had discovered weight loss for the emotions.

~Kiss of the Butterfly~

"ARE YOU CLAUSTROPHOBIC?" asked the technician.

"Nope."

The MRI gulped me whole. My breath lodged in my chest and my heart raced to its rescue. *Breathe. Just breathe. It's too tight. The walls are too close. I need space. I need to sit up. I need to see. Breathe.* I rethought my response to his question.

"You doing okay?" came the technician's voice through the speaker.

"Yep, I'm good," My words squeezed through pursed lips. The deeper I breathed, the more I settled into the chamber. Another breath and another, until suddenly a jackhammer.

My eighteen-month-old daughter liked special kisses at bedtime: rubbing noses in a polar bear kiss or the soft, nearly imperceptible flutter of eyelashes on cheek of a butterfly kiss. Bending over her crib to deliver my kisses sent searing pain down from my low back to hide behind my knees, forcing them to buckle. After years of relapses of pain and weakness in my legs, Aunt Joyce convinced me to book a diagnostic exam to reveal the extent of damage to my spine.

As I lay still, the near-deafening pounding and rhythmic rattling of the MRI chamber hypnotically numbing me to sleep, an email slipped into the inbox on my laptop sitting on the kitchen table back home. Like the butterfly effect, wings silently flapping, the email gently initiated a change of weather about to move into my life. Unknown to the sender or me, a storm brewed, carrying the potential of transformation, if I could weather it.

Silence woke me. The MRI spit me back out. I dressed and returned to the reception desk where my CD copy of the results awaited. An appointment with the back specialist was months away. Health care in Canada was free but sometimes you had to wait for it. The CD proved useless to me. But a qualified practitioner could read it. Someone like Aunt Joyce.

I headed to her clinic. Joyce led me into her treatment room and loaded the CD into her computer. She pointed out a massive herniation in one of my discs, a tear in the disc above that, desiccation in the upper discs, degeneration of the facet joints responsible for side to side movement of the torso, and moderate stenosis, the condition responsible for the hunching-over seen most often in the elderly. All of this on an already scoliotic spine.

I had known for years about the scoliosis, but I didn't realize it was a double curve, a subtle S. My spine not only curved but also twisted. Basically, instead of a straight spine, my primary support for my body resembled a ride at Disneyland. Except the rides at Disneyland were in better condition. S for spine, S for scoliosis, S for Stephanie.

I listened intently, unable to digest the information. I knew, however, Joyce's help gave me a jump on recovery, and I could begin to adjust my lifestyle immediately and accordingly. She spoke frankly. "The images are not what I like to see in someone your age."

Great. If this is me at thirty-seven, what will sixty-seven look like? I'm screwed.

She was right to prompt me to have the test done. Seeing the size of the bulge in my disc and the shape of my spine was a wakeup call. I'd have lived in denial another four years, perhaps longer, expecting my body to return to its former glory.

Aunt Joyce made recommendations: swimming and yoga in lieu of running and high impact sports, no weight training or any compressive activities. She even told me not to walk on pavement for prolonged periods of time if I could avoid it.

Get your head around it. I coached myself. *And get going.*

"I can beat anything," I said aloud on the drive home. I didn't have the wisdom at the time to know that healing wasn't about *beating* anything, but about making peace with something.

I returned home, set my CD on the kitchen table and flipped open the lid on my laptop, ready to dive into all available research on my injury and formulate a plan. At the bottom of my screen, the little red circle with the number inside dangled like candy. I clicked on the icon to reveal an email from my dear friend Anna: an invitation to join a year of yoga in her small hamlet, starting March. I read the message but it might as well have been written in pig Latin.

My pep-talk on the way home had failed. I closed my laptop and cried for three days. I had a vision of supermom, playing sports with my kids, learning to snowboard with them, and waterskiing, hiking, climbing, and weight training into my nineties. All of it crumbled around me.

What have I done to myself? Was it the years of weight-training? Then the victim came; *why me?* I'd done everything *right*. I ate right. I exercised. I helped others eat right and exercise.

Not only was training my livelihood, it was my life. Most people complained about not being able to drag themselves into the gym; I had difficulty dragging myself *out* of the gym. I always took the stairs instead of the elevator, and was game for any new sport. What was I supposed to do? Aunt Joyce had recommended swimming, but I hated public pools and gagged at the thought of a chlorine-laden facial. I enjoyed yoga as a stretch, but it was no match for incline leg press and wide-grip pull ups. And no running?

Sitting on my living room floor, I tried to appreciate the good in my life, that I didn't have a more serious condition, that my family and I were healthy, but I couldn't stuff my emotions by comparing my situation to someone worse off. I had to deal with my depression, with the grief and the anger. The last pieces of my vibrant self turned to dust, and, mixed with my tears, soiled the living room rug. *Who puts a cream-coloured carpet in a house with small children anyway?*

We never chose the carpet. We had bought the house from the original owners. Over the years, I had scrubbed black felt, spilled potted soil, cat puke, chai tea and tread-mill grease from the carpet. I'm sure I'll get the drippings of my life's dreams out too.

The bipolar nature of my coping skills continued and a gust of determination lifted me to my feet. *There has to be a way to clean this up: to heal the injury and repair the damage. There is no way I am going to live anything less than an active, healthy life with my family. I'll find a way. Maybe Anna's email is part of that way.* At least I could feed my appetite for exercise with the intensive days of yoga.

I returned to the invite for a closer look. The email for the yoga journey outlined the year organized by chakras. I knew little about the chakra system, only that it consisted of seven energy centers located at different points in the body and that various health conditions corresponded to them. I gleaned this from a book, *Why People Don't Heal and How They Can* by Caroline Myss. I had thumbed through it years earlier, loaned to me by Aunt Joyce after my injury.

Seven chakras. One chakra retreat day every forty days. One year in yoga. Well, most of a year. Participation required regularly scheduled full days away from the kids.

The cost required justification. I waffled back and forth for days.

"How great would it be to dive into a year of yoga *and* spend that year together?" Anna's whispered excitement raised the hairs on my arms. It had been months since we'd spoken on the phone. Both mothers, Anna with a toddler and me with a preschooler and a baby, we struggled to find time together since children. I'm not sure if she whispered because her daughter Kayla was napping or because our topic of discussion was too fragile to speak aloud. "We can connect again, as friends, outside of children and partners and the chaos of life. I've already signed up, Steph."

Meeting every forty days would require Steve to look after the kids. I cringed at the thought of asking him to make that commitment for an entire year. I found all sorts of excuses, yet I returned again and again to the invitation. The timing was uncanny — on the heels of my MRI results when I was faced with a major lifestyle change. Being with the yoga group would allow me to take a day to myself — no kids or husband. I wanted that time. I needed it. However, many shades of guilt coloured my decision, along with concern for my kids' welfare.

No one met their needs as well as I did, or so I believed. They required a special diet and without me controlling all the details, things could fall apart. There were nap schedules, dressing for the weather and potential injuries or illness. How could thinking about leaving make my stomach churn, while not taking time away deepened the elevens between my brows? Where was the happy medium? Was balance bullshit? Still, the invitation loomed large in my thoughts.

"Yeah, of course, Hon, whatever you need."

I had expected a contentious conversation with Steve.

Since kids, time as a couple was non-existent, let alone time to ourselves. It meant the other had to put in even more effort. In a time period my cousin likes to refer to as B.C. (before children), Steve and I watched every movie that made it to the theatre, even midnight screenings.

Steve introduced me to his favourite cult classic movies like *Bad Taste* and *This is Spinal Tap*, where, in a famous scene, an amplifier goes from zero to eleven instead of ten. Nigel's character says, "... if we need that extra push over the cliff, you know what we do?" Marty's character responds, "Put it up to eleven."

Since kids, in order for Steve or I to have time to ourselves, the other had to *put it up to eleven*.

Steve's support secured my decision. I replied to the email, sent a cheque and committed to a year in yoga.

"New beginnings are often disguised as painful endings."
~Lao Tzu

PART I

ROOT CHAKRA

FOUNDATION

To establish a solid foundation,
sometimes you have to dig up the old
and lay down the new.

1

STUMBLING AROUND IN THE DARK

I didn't sleep that night, not because the kids woke or the husband snored. I didn't sleep because I worried the kids *might* wake or the husband *might* snore and I needed to be up by five o'clock and out of the house by six.

I swung my legs over the edge of my warm bed and pushed off the duvet. My spine cried out. I eased from the bed in an attempt to mitigate both the pain radiating across my back and the squeaking of the mattress frame.

The alarm clock threatened only minutes until five. Nervousness combined with anticipation of the day's events prevented me from crawling back under the covers and passing out. I kept it together long enough to slip quietly around the foot of the bed and alongside my sleeping husband to disarm the alarm clock. I couldn't risk disturbing slumbering bodies that might result in a cranky day for them and interfere with my quick escape from the house.

My eyes stung. I shuffled down the stairs and into the bathroom where my clothes and makeup waited, carefully laid out the night before. Leaning on the cool porcelain of the pedestal sink, I brushed my teeth and applied the standard blush, liner, shadow and gloss. I pulled my dark hair into a stylish ponytail, bangs swept across my brow.

I stared into the mirror. It didn't reflect my depleted mood and body. I felt frail but with my mask in place, appeared beautiful and strong. I tried to hurry, but my body had one gear: tired. I had packed most items the previous night: yoga mat, books, notepad, pen, a second pair of pants, extra socks, hiking boots and a picture of my family for the altar, as per the group email instructions.

I popped two slices of bread in the toaster while I laid out a few last minute items. I slapped peanut butter and jam on the toast, placed one piece atop the other, sandwich style, wrapped it up in paper towel and set it on the back step while I loaded my gear into the trunk of the car. I drove west through the dark, down the highway, eating my breakfast.

Thirty minutes later, I pulled into the small hamlet and parked my car in the empty lot of the main shopping plaza. I stepped out of my vehicle and stretched my arms over head to wake my body. Blood rushed my spine in comfort. I took a deep breath of country air, relieved to be out of the city and in the quiet hours of the hamlet.

Two vehicles crept onto the lot and parked a couple aisles away, no movement from the occupants. The air stood still, heavy with darkness. I waited for someone to step out and join me. I took a deep breath and decided to layer up while I had the time.

I balanced on one foot, leaning against the car to mitigate the pain while I removed each rubber boot, pulled on my second pair of pants and stepped into my hiking shoes. Still no movement from the other cars. *What next?* I wanted a familiar face or at least better instructions.

I pulled on my jacket and gloves as a large, dark truck

cozied up alongside me. A door opened and a couple women in the backseat leaned over and invited me to join them. It was like a strange scene from a spy novel.

I complied with the orders I'd received in the email. I grabbed my gear, locked my car and jumped into the truck. I introduced myself to the other passengers, unable to make out faces in the dark. The warm cab smelled of new vehicle and men's cologne — an inviting combination of wood and spice. The soft orange glow of the dash lights, and the scent and warmth in the truck's cabin, provided strange reassurance as my thoughts pointed out that I was in the backseat of an unfamiliar truck driven by a man I didn't know, in the dark early morning hours, heading to who knows where.

I didn't *feel* scared. My body felt cozy and comfortable, only my mind pointed out the myriad of reasons I *should* feel scared. I stared out the window into the dark. Where was Anna? She got me into this.

Nearly fifteen years earlier, before husbands and kids, Anna had become a friend when I'd forgotten what it was like to have one. Several years of my life had been marred by destructive relationships and resultant low self-esteem. At twenty-three years old, I had landed a job in an art gallery in the small tourist town of Banff, Alberta. The upscale shop offered original art, sculpture and artisan jewelry. The owner reminded me of Katherine Hepburn in her later years: gracious and graceful, despite her trembling hands. It was a comfortable place for me to land — an inviting environment filled with elegant art and civilized people, the most civilized of whom was my dear friend, Anna.

We opened shop each morning, selecting from the stunning array of bijoux and bobbles to accessorize our well-assembled ensembles. We chose the day's music: *What a difference a day makes...* Dinah Washington's sultry voice crooned through the gallery as we sipped apple-spiced tea and gazed upon the Rocky Mountains through the large gallery windows, awaiting the arrival of the diverse, well-heeled tourist clientele.

I loved the atmosphere of the shop, the slower pace, the pleasantries and the company of the ladies who worked there. I particularly enjoyed the artist receptions where Anna and I dressed up, put on the dog as well as our jewels. We'd make silly faces at each other, sticking out our tongues when neither clients nor bosses were looking. We behaved like two young girls in church expected to act like ladies yet taking great delight in covert rebellion.

"You know he was on acid when he painted that," Anna whispered.

"What?" I burst, caught off guard by her comment.

She chuckled. "He just told me that himself."

"Well," I cocked my head sideways to consider the large painting. "I guess you'd *have* to be to work with *those* colours."

I needed to feel like a child again, innocent and playful. I'd given up much of it while I'd given up my self-worth in the preceding years that led me to Banff and to Anna: years of leaving home for school, life as a starving student, post-secondary burnout and diving into a destructive relationship in search of reprieve. Looking back, those impressionable young adult years were fleeting and foreign, yet felt definitive at the time. We are not condemned to be who we once were: poor judges of men, starving students and college drop-outs.

Our paths took us in different directions over the years; mine led back to the city and Anna's to the small hamlet. After nearly fifteen years of roving friendship, we always reunited in delight of one another's company while we caught up on adventures and plans. *Sister cats*, we called ourselves, the name borrowed from a humorous birthday card Anna gave me one year.

When Anna emailed me about the year in yoga with a group of strangers in her hamlet of Bragg Creek, I had been apprehensive about joining, but her participation reassured me that I had not embarked on the journey alone. Nothing to worry about; sister cat would be right there with me ... *but where was she?*

I looked for her as the truck slowed and pulled off the road, then parked behind several other vehicles. As I stepped out of the cocoon of the truck's cabin and back into the cold darkness, I made out the images of others gathered at an opening in the trees near the road. I approached the group and recognized the voice of my dear friend visiting with others at the trailhead. Anna and I hugged briefly before a woman began to address the group. She spoke in a gentle voice, yet a tone that attempted to gain control over the small cluster of people that chatted like chickadees on a cold morning.

"Please walk in silence from here on," the woman said.

It was difficult to determine how many of us assembled in the dark and unfamiliar territory. We began our hike to the first clearing on the hillside. The air hung still and the snow crunched loudly under our feet in the early morning hours. The endless dark sky gave a sense that I was wandering into vast new territory.

We approached the clearing. The woman introduced Stephen, a Qigong Master, though it occurred to me she'd never formally introduced herself. Stephen gathered us in a circle.

"Place your feet in a wide stance and gently bend your knees. Relax your upper body."

It was a March Alberta morning. Chilly. I tried to focus on the exercises and not my cold hands. What happened to yoga?

I followed the breathing and visualizations, drawing energy from the earth up the inside of my legs and back down, my eyes fixed shut. Unsure I felt any energy other than trembling from the cold, I followed Stephen's guidance, imagining energy moving up, feet apart, knees slightly bent to accommodate the culmination of the energy in an invisible seat nestled just under my pelvis. I couldn't feel the seat or the culmination of energy but I held the idea in my head, wondering if the others enjoyed perching on an invisible stool of qi.[1]

As we finished, I opened my eyes, surprised to see my surroundings glowing in the early light of morning. The snow-covered foothills shone a luminescent blue as night yielded to day. We lingered in silence until the familiar voice of Alora broke through. She was to be our guide for our early morning hike and yoga for the forthcoming year.

"Come closer," Alora instructed the group.

I turned to see her in the dim light for the first time. A petite blonde with tiny features and long, straight hair stood in the snow, under layers of winter wear. Removing her mittens, she pulled a folded sheet of paper from her pocket. Hands shaking, she read aloud a First Nation's prophecy. A poem of sorts. Instructions for living. A survival guide, perhaps.

"You have been telling people that this is the Eleventh Hour, now you must go back and tell the people that this is the Hour. And there are things to be considered...

Where are you living?

What are you doing?

What are your relationships?

Are you in right relation?
Where is your water?
Know your garden.
It is time to speak your truth.
Create your community.
Be good to each other.
And do not look outside yourself for your leader..."[2]

The prophecy felt important, not necessarily to our first gathering, but encompassing the nature of the year's journey ahead. A couple lines sounded foreboding, something about clinging to the shore and suffering. Although I didn't understand it all, the poem resonated with me.

After the invocation, we continued our hike up the trail in silent walking meditation, crunching snow under our feet, the only sound. Dawn's light revealed our path through the gently treed winter landscape. I watched the boots of the person in front of me.

A distance naturally formed between the group members as each made their way in their own cadence up the hill. I wandered along, led by my thoughts. The sky appeared between the leafless trees. Previously trodden snow formed a packed and often slippery layer under the fresh white powder. I tried to keep my footing steady, in line with the existing tread marks of hikers before us. I tried to meditate, and although meditation itself was not new to me, moving meditation proved foreign. I simply enjoyed the walk, the view, the sounds, the fresh air and the opportunity to create warmth through movement. Maybe that *was* moving meditation.

The view from the top justified each and every teeth-chattering step. The west and south revealed the silhouette of the Canadian Rocky Mountains in the near distance. Silent giants, still asleep in the early morning light. Communities of near-leafless birch trees on the top of Two Pine Hill camouflaged the east and north like sentinels. A gently sloping crest, maybe fifteen feet wide, offered our group a place to gather and rest. We all gravitated toward the west, claimed spots to sit and continue our silent contemplation. Happy I wore my snow pants, I I gently lowered myself to the ground, crossed my legs and arms for extra warmth, and tucked my gloved hands into my armpits.

"Contemplate what you want as your focus." Alora's voice sailed over the hill top. "Something to draw into your life or let go of ... to hold in your consciousness for our inquiries together over our year in yoga."

Family.

Where did that come from? It felt like someone else spoke inside my head. My motivation to join the year in yoga stemmed from my back injury. Healing the injury seemed the most logical intention for my year, or at least my own self care, yet the first word to surface was *family*. I didn't even know where it came from. It tethered itself in my mind. I had come for my spine.

Family.

Why Family? It must be important because it was all I could hear. I began to excavate its origin. What was this tug-of-war between me and family?

My kids had changed my life dramatically. Most days, I felt as though I was stumbling through fog. Balance ceased to exist. I had imagined a gentle transition from proud, beaming pregnant lady to peaceful, wise and nurtured new mother. Instead, the earthquake of motherhood left me feeling sleep-deprived, defensive, unsupported, unsure, overly protective and fumbling around in unfamiliar terri-tory while trying to project the persona of a perfect parent. Raising kids, thriving in a marriage, personally fulfilled and finding happiness in it all, seemed elusive, if not impossible — fleeting and surreal at best.

Utter exhaustion overshadowed happiness. Both kids suffered discomfort and sleep issues due to food intolerances. I received little help in identifying and rectifying their issues. In fact, I often battled against the common opinion of doctors and specialists, fighting a righteous uphill battle to find the root of my children's pain. One thing propelled me: the burning inner knowing that there indeed *was* a root and that once I found it, I could rip it from the ground and we could all rest easier.

With Michael five-years-old and Khali nearly two, I had found the answers I sought but had no ability to maintain my well-being while working to restore theirs, no idea of my sacrifice. Or, perhaps, as a mother, I believed that's what moms did, sacrifice. With the root of the issue known, dietary adjustments made and both kids sleeping well, my adrenaline subsided, as did the crusade that had compelled me, and I realized how depleted I'd become.

My relationship with Steve was also not as I imagined. We struggled to find energy to simply manage the kids and work. A game of *who put in the most hours* played out in our marriage. Bitter tones and annoyed glances replaced lively conversation as our form of communication. The most daunting aspect was that I couldn't tell where I fit into the picture: what *I* wanted out of life: what inspired me: what brought *me* joy. No longer an active participant, I went through the motions of my life mostly tired, resentful and passionless.

"Write down your focus." Alora's whisper halted my train of thought. She handed me a slip of paper and a pencil. I quietly thanked her, removed my gloves and jotted down FAMILY, solidifying my focus before I changed my mind. I watched as she approached each member of our group, reverently, trying not to disturb their reflective states. I returned my gaze to the mountains. Cradling the Rockies' chiseled chin in its hand, the rising sun slowly turned the mountain's face to meet mine.

After what seemed like hours that morning, and years of my life before, stumbling around in the dark, the emerging light of the sun brought clarity to the previously colourless forms around me. The shades of blue morphed into yellows like a time-lapsed video of a sunflower blossoming. The bright, open sky starkly contrasted the enshrouding darkness; a sobering sight.

The warmth of the sun's rays reached me. I turned my face away from the mountain range and toward the glow. The texture of the partly peeled and weathered white bark on the birch trees caught my eye. A few lifeless yet tenacious leaves grasped their branches, having refused to drop with the others in the fall; instead they had survived the long winter months to cheer the sun's return. How did some hold fast while others surrendered to the changing weather?

I turned back to stare at the sunlit giants, the mountains' features fully accentuated by the light. Snow cradled heavy in their valley. Sharp peaks exposed blue-grey rock dotted with white where the snow found ledges to rest. I deeply inhaled the cold, fresh air.

"Could you all gather in a circle, please?" Alora's voice once again broke the silence and pulled me from my sensory trance. I took my time getting back on my feet. We gathered around, able to see each other and introduce ourselves for the first time. A celebratory feeling emerged among group members. People smiled, said hello, shared a laugh or excited raised eyebrows. The morning's experience strangely unified us, even in silence. Perhaps because of it.

Upon clearly seeing Alora, I realized I had met her ten years earlier, perhaps longer ago, certainly before kids. I had met her as Lorraine, but she had taken on the spiritual name, Alora, through her yoga training. Anna had invited me to attend an intimate yoga class in the basement of Alora's home. I remembered her house: a log home, ornate with silky throw cushions, statues of ancient deities, and Eastern masks and paintings hanging on the walls.

I remembered thinking how Anna's teacher exuded the yogic lifestyle, in living quarters as well as mannerisms. She had greeted us warmly and spoke lovingly to three beautiful little blonde girls — a stunning family. The yoga she guided us through felt organic, nourishing and deeply relaxing. The pace and postures revealed a layer absent from traditional exercise.

I suddenly understood Anna's desire for the year in yoga and the community guided by Alora. Anna recently reconnected with Alora for weekly yoga classes and had told me about the impact of those classes on her life. She said she felt changed.

I watched Alora in the new light as she spoke to us, purposefully. Her smooth voice quivered occasionally either from nerves or the cold, perhaps both. She looked older than that first time we'd met. I glanced at Anna across the circle of people. She was striking. Her shoulder-length brown hair escaped her toque. Her brilliant blue eyes and thick dark brows gave expression to her clear skin. The cold air swept blush onto her cheeks. I thought how we *all* looked older, Anna, Alora and me. Maturity settled around the corners of our eyes and the edges of our smiles.

I didn't feel more mature. The youngest of the three of us, in my late thirties, I still felt twenty-three: the driven, tenacious, girl who joked and laughed in the Banff art gallery with Anna. Well, I didn't actually *feel* that way; more accurately, I *expected* to feel that way. The memory lingered in me as if I'd never transitioned from that place in my life; the experiences, ripe and vivid, were firmly entrenched in my mind.

The past ten years had come and gone and I hadn't really lived them. I owned the memories yet most of them contained little colour or richness. Of course, I recalled vividly my wedding and the birth of my children. It was hard to sleep through those monumental experiences. The rest lingered like a dream, and I expected to wake any moment, with all the vitality and beauty of my twenty-three-year-old form, only wiser.

I surveyed the group. With the exception of Alora's daughter, we all wore the mask of maturity, perhaps fifteen of us, mainly women. I guessed the age range from thirty-five to fifty-five as I panned the faces of the group wondering about each person's motivation to be there. Many appeared to know one another. Most lived in the hamlet and, I assumed, attended Alora's regular yoga classes.

I never considered the possibility of a mixed gathering. The male component drew my defences. Although exposed in the bright light of day, concerned about judgment and scrutiny from the others, I took comfort in hiding inside my layers of winter clothing.

Alora requested our slips of paper and we handed them to her for burning, intentions to be released to the universe for fulfillment over the coming year. She crouched over a small bowl filled with our individual statements and struck a match, which quickly extinguished. She struck another, holding her hand around the tentative flame as it, too, failed to ignite the papers. She tried a third match as we stood, waiting and watching, pressing our collective bodies as a shield against the faint breeze, in expectation of ignition. A March Alberta foothills morning proved less than conducive to conjure fire.

Alora collected the papers from the pot and placed them in her bag on the ground. "I'll take these home to burn," she said.

I had placed my family on that paper and felt uneasy with it in her hands. I wasn't sure which was more odd, the feeling of concern over leaving my family in her hands, or the bizarre idea of releasing our intentions into the universe through burning.

Gathered in a circle once more, Alora introduced another guest facilitator, Lil, who had spent time with a First Nations community in the southern United States. I found it difficult to guess her age, for her long grey hair, pulled into a loosely braided ponytail, suggested advanced years. Her youthful smile and movements intimated she was younger than she appeared. She wore a multi-coloured poncho of sorts, woven and cozy looking, and she shared stories of time spent on Indigenous lands with Elders and their wisdom.

She held up a rattle, round with a straight handle and painted in blues, reds and white. She turned to the east, asking us to follow. She shook the rattle. It answered, echoing a rattlesnake's warning through the valley. She spoke aloud to the sky. Calling out the names of animal spirits, she asked for their blessings, protection and guidance. She turned to the south and we followed. She called on more animals, repeating in the west and north.

The rhythmic echo of the rattle revived me while Lil's words intrigued me. Did their poetic flow result from practice or had they emerged in the moment? The ceremony opened our year of self exploration, asking the four directions and their various spirits to guide us and protect us on the journey.

Lil fell silent. As did the rattle. Only when my shoulders resumed shivering did I realize that they had stopped during the invocation.

"Take a deep breath in and let it go." Alora reclaimed the group. "I have one more practice for you. Everyone put your right hand in the circle. You put your right hand in, you put your right hand out..."

Yes, Alora led us in the famous self discovery tool known as the *Hokey Pokey*. The finale? A crescendo of wiggling backsides pointed into the middle of the circle and at one another. My backside wiggled ever so gingerly so as not to disturb my spine. *Shake it all about.* Any remnants of unfamiliarity between group members dissipated as we laughed and snorted our way through the ending of the song. We gathered our things and made our way down the mountain, sister cat and I, finally free to talk.

2

THESE ROOTS SMELL FAMILIAR

I followed Anna's car in my own down the highway and onto a rural tree-lined road. She slowed and her signal light flashed. She'd found it. A hand-carved log sign spanned the entrance of the driveway: *Sacred Forest Lodge*.

I drove up the lane, flooded by memories of life growing up in the country: horseback riding across the crop-less fields of early spring and late fall; new batches of spring kittens wrestling in the sun in front of the barn; snowmobiling under moonlit skies — headlights off as snow illuminated my way; skating on the slough; family picnics in the trees, spitting watermelon seeds and hurtling rinds at my older sister and cousins.

I opened the car door and smelled the earthiness of horses. The sunlight sparkled off the snow in front of the red barns: instant therapy. Trees hugged the property and lined the pastures. A creek, whose steady flow kept ice from concealing it, streaked through the main pasture behind the cabin. Horses, chickens, and several cats called Sacred Forest home, as did countless deer, birds, an owl, and even a beaver. The main residents, however, consisted of a husband, wife, and two children: a boy and a girl.

Gabriella and her husband, Luca, originally hailed from Italy. They owned the picturesque property, had improved many of its buildings, and operated Sacred Forest Lodge. They rented the various rooms and cabins to families and individuals seeking nature and retreat. They also happened to be participants in our year of yoga.

A long wooden porch greeted me. In the entry hall past the front door, I removed my boots and hung my jacket. Directly ahead, a steep ladder lined a log wall. I grabbed hold of the wooden rail and climbed into a loft. A vaulted ceiling, half-moon window and colourful floor mandala, hand-painted by Luca, crowned the cabin.

Back downstairs, I walked past an antique stove and large dining table which filled only half of the immense kitchen, the heartbeat of the cabin, where women were busy chatting and making tea. I explored each of the rooms like a home buyer happening upon a juicy listing. The attention to detail displayed by Gabriella and Luca proved a testament to their love for the land, nature and art: from the hand-carved and painted bed posts to the fluffy comforters and overstuffed pillows, to fresh eggs gathered each morning for their guests, the couple took pride in Sacred Forest.

My favourite room was the massive sunroom where we set our bags and placed our mats in preparation for yoga practice. An obvious addition to the original 1945 cabin, natural light poured in through a wall of windows lining the south and the sliding glass doors on the west and east walls. The vaulted wood ceiling boasted a level of rectangular skylights on either side. I felt at home in the big bright room, aglow with morning rays.

A hot cup of tea welcomed us after the sunrise hike. I

felt as though I'd already lived an entire day. Muffins and orange slices filled the counter: energy for our first yoga practice as a group. I placed my mat in the sunroom by the screen door, which I cracked open an inch. Sparrows prattled away in the tall evergreens.

The strength of the March sun's rays overcame the icy air filtering through the screen door. I stretched out like a cat on my mat, drenched in sunlight. I looked forward to a vigorous yoga practice.

Somewhere along the way I had claimed training as my identity. I craved it, even if it was destroying my body. The full day of yoga was the dessert that satisfied my sweet tooth while keeping the dentist at bay. If weights were no longer part of my diet, perhaps I could indulge in extra helpings of yoga.

"We'll be on our mats until lunch." Alora rolled her mat out near the doorway to the living room. "I have other inquiries planned for our afternoon."

Whoa. What? Not even a half-day of yoga? I needed to tax my muscles and fatigue my body in the familiar fashion I had conducted for nearly twenty years. I decided to crank up the intensity.

"The first chakra is located at the base of the spine," Alora said as she stood at the front of her mat. "This energy centre is red."

She continued to expound the encyclopedia of first chakra while she led us through a series of postures specific to root chakra: *muladhara*, Sanskrit for *root place*.

"Foods that feed root chakra are root vegetables, ginger, mushrooms, and red-coloured foods like tomatoes, strawberries, red apples and pomegranates." Alora had us in mountain pose: tall and strong on our mats, unwavering.

"First chakra represents Earth and our connection to her."

Interesting ... referring to the planet as "her." It felt strange to me but appeared important to Alora and others in the group, so I opted in. It would take some getting used to, seeing the planet as more than a home for trees, water and animals, but a living entity of her own: a being.

Root chakra encompassed all things Earth and primal: foundation, security, survival, food, shelter, individual identity and our connection to Nature. Discovering my place on the planet and my connection to Earth both tied into first chakra. Questioning if I felt safe and supported in life, with strong roots and a firm base, gave me a sense of muladhara.

Earth postures of warrior I and II, pigeon pose, low lunge and savasana provided a sense of grounding, focus and solidity. They encouraged my body to yield to the floor and to Earth, allowing her complete support. The most fundamental of the chakras, root chakra held the potential to strengthen my base of support from which I would grow over the year. It was up to me to decide, through my work in first chakra, how strong that base would become.

We found our way into the standing poses, holding for long periods, legs shaking, muscles burning. Alora read aloud an affirmation and we repeated it, followed by a deep, resounding, from the base of our spine, primal release: *Yeeeesssss!* Well, some members' releases were more primal than others. It took effort on my part to release the hounds. It reminded me of the overly dramatic moaning and groaning that often occurred on the weight room floor.

"I am here, fully experiencing my body ... yessss," she read, "I am taking responsibility for my life ... yessss."

Each affirmation sank into our consciousness as we sank deeper into the pose, repeating the words louder and louder. Voices strained as we struggled to keep our bodies upright and continue to breathe. The energy of the group intensified and heat filled the room. Moisture gathered in my hairline and pooled along the straps of my tank top.

I held the pose for the duration, not giving in to lowering to the ground like several others. I obstinately held, legs quivering. I resisted the urge to lower, not because I trusted my legs to support me as the ground supported my legs, but because I fed off the intensity of the exercise and my appearance of strength to the others. I supported myself because it kept me safe, *I* kept me safe, and I had worked hard for many years for that strength, to support myself.

"Aaaaaaaaaaaaahhhhhhhh," Yvonne sighed almost orgasmically as she lowered her body to the floor.

I held. My legs shook. I knew survival. I had struggled to survive as a young adult: as a starving student delivering pizza to pay my rent, only to find it barely covered the gas. I spent much of my twenties in fight-or-flight mode, determined to take care of myself, too proud to ask for help and making one bad decision after another.

Used to the duelling egos found on the weight room floors, in confrontational relationships, and around the boardroom table at morning marketing meetings during my years in the corporate world, I found myself lacking in the ability to relate in the casual group setting. The easy nature and openness of my fellow yoga members put me off my game. I approached the experience from a place of competition rather than camaraderie. I had lost the basic ability to communicate authentically and naturally with people: no strategy, no motive, no objective, simply myself, comfortable in my own skin.

I didn't see myself through my thirty-seven-year-old eyes. I viewed myself as I imagined others saw me, and my imagination conjured negative remarks and judgments that triggered my defences before any actual attack mounted. I was always on guard for what may be coming, another way to protect myself. Force fields raised as the intensity of the pose increased. Like a yoga pissing match, I persevered in the posture, oblivious to the fact that the match was not between me and the others, but me and my ego.

I had no idea that everything that emerged during my poses reflected the very nature of root chakra. At a fundamental level, I didn't feel safe and I didn't feel supported. I was stuck in a pattern of fight or flight that left me unable to relax.

That morning, yoga shone a light on how I thought, felt and acted around others, the environments in which I had previously conditioned myself to survive, and the importance that others perceive me as strong and independent. Others in the group seemed more relaxed, more themselves, easy smiles, easy breathing, yielding contently to the floor when their bodies signalled enough. No one else's outfit looked like a power suit: black, fitted and well-coordinated.

Sandra, with her British accent and wit, and her stylish short brown hair, swaggered about the sunroom looking perfectly at home, with her sweet smile and clever quips. Thoughts flooded my brain competing for space in my head and pressing on the seams of my skull, which started to hurt more than my back. I jotted the remaining affirmations in my journal so I could practice alone, later, removed from the distracting group dynamic.

I lay flat on my back, eyes closed in savasana, yoga's final resting pose. Corpse pose. Play dead. *Sparrows' chirping... chirping... chirping... reminds me of ringing.*

Fifteen years earlier, I had heard the fire alarms go off in my Calgary high rise apartment suite and remained in bed.

A string of false alarms had cried wolf too many times that week and I decided to sleep that one out. The firemen who banged on my door had other ideas. They informed me of the fine for not vacating the building.

At that time, I managed one of a group of restaurants owned by a friend's husband. Appreciative of the job, I struggled with my boss' bipolar personality: the kindest man one minute, tearing a strip off me the next. I never knew which version of him I would meet on any given day. Each work day ended with me driving around the city, collecting the daily deposits from the various restaurants and delivering them downtown to my boss at two in the morning. I would then drag my tired self into my apartment, order Greek for two-thirty dinner and wash it down with a half bottle of red wine. I was twenty-two.

My late hours at work forced a three o'clock bedtime. The fire alarm early that morning left me sitting on the cool cement curb, feet on the avenue and head in my hands at seven. I cracked. I started laughing. All of it was hilarious: the woman smuggling her cat in her oversized purse, people in pyjamas on the sidewalk, the four fire trucks parked on the street, the twenty-five flights of stairs that had become my regular early morning workout. The ridiculousness that was my life. Hysterical.

Maybe it was the lack of sleep. Maybe I was so exhausted I was delusional, and in that altered state, I didn't care anymore. Maybe the stars and the moon had aligned with Uranus.

In that time on the curb, nearly an entire hour, in a tiny mob of disheveled strangers who slept only feet from one another, something inside me snapped. Something needed to change. *Everything* needed to change: my job, my living arrangement, my sleep, the people I surrounded myself with. Young and single, nothing kept me there. I stood in the sun in my pyjamas and hoody and called my employer from the payphone on the corner.

"I am *not* coming in today." My tone was non-negotiable. "I am taking a personal day."

The next call went to my mom. "I'm coming home."

I drove the ninety-minutes to Mom's office. From the desk next to hers, I searched the wanted ads, typed resumés and faxed them to potential employers. It was convenient to have all that office equipment at my disposal since Mom and Dad didn't even own a computer.

Within a couple hours I received a call from an art gallery in Banff. The Monday morning interview for the Assistant Manager position afforded me a weekend of reprieve at home with my parents. I slept, lounged on the deck in the sunshine, watched movies and ate Mom's comfort food — good farm food: meat and potatoes. We devoured Burnt Almond bars and drank Nestlé iced tea, the powdered kind that you mix with water.

Come Monday morning, I drove straight from Red Deer to Banff, nearly three hours, for my interview. I chose the back country roads over the main highway. I had forgotten how beautiful the countryside was, and it appeared even more alive that day; roadside poplars cheered me on as wild grasses waved.

I landed the position and continued my drive into Calgary, to my job, where I promptly and proudly gave notice. I was fuelled by restful sleep, chocolate, mountain air, and the chance for change.

Within the week, I had packed up what little my apartment held of my life. The night before my move, I hit the biggest country bar in the city with a dear friend: the wife of my ex-boss. Poetic. It was Stampede week and the place was jumping. We lived on the dance floor, no shortage of two-stepping partners during the Greatest Outdoor Show on Earth. Soaked in sweat, we poured ourselves into a cab at two in the morning and I landed at my box-filled apartment to order pizza. I abandoned the leftovers on the counter and passed out for the last time in that space. *Fuck you, fire alarm.*

My Aussie brother-in-law arrived with my mom, dad and sister at seven to help with the move. "Mmmm, pizza," he said through a mouthful.

"Um, that's been sitting out all night," I replied.

"And?" he mumbled as he grabbed another slice.

I uprooted myself to start over in the small tourist town. Truthfully, I had no roots in the city. They couldn't penetrate the concrete. I could tell Mom and Dad were nervous to leave me there, but I was ready for change. Sharing a large house with seven quiet, young, Japanese girls who spoke little English and cleaned often, proved to be the gentle and calm environment I needed. Sitting on the front steps of the great old home, a giant pine tree for company, surrounded by mountains, feet on the ground, I had escaped the crazy and found comfort in the quiet.

"Gently begin to wiggle fingers and toes," Alora's voice woke me from my death pose. "Roll onto your right side and rest a moment. When you're ready, come to sitting on your mat."

Easier said than done. How about I just roll around on the floor for a while? When I was up, I was good. When I was down, I was good. It was during the transition from lying down to standing, that things could go sideways. I pulled my core tight, took a deep breath and pressed my upper body upright.

My nervous system was a frazzled watchman, on constant guard, paranoid of the next attack. I would never see it coming. I'd hope I was safe but the pain conditioned me to anticipate the worst. Used to the ache in my muscles, my mind probed the pain in my low back for signs of imminent lock-up, prepared to nose-dive if necessary. My spine obliged and stacked one vertebrae on top of the other. *Yessssssssss.*

"We'll continue our practice with alternate nostril breathing." Alora brought her right hand to her face. "Bring your index and middle fingers of your right hand to press against your third eye ... the space between your brows. Gently press your thumb into the side of your right nostril, just below the bone ... not the fat, fleshy part."

I followed her lead.

"Now, inhale through the left nostril. Draw the breath slow and deep into the body ... hold. Press your ring finger into the side of the left nostril and remove your thumb. Exhale long and slow from the right nostril ... stay. Inhale through the right ... pause. Switch fingers and exhale left. *Nadi shodhana,* Sanskrit for purification of nadis, or channels."

My nostril kept sticking to itself when I released my finger. Held by snot glue, my nose whistled when I forced the air in and out of my congested nasal passages. I wanted to get up and blow it, make it stop. I wasn't about to disrupt the process. I nose-whistled on.

We continued the cycle. The congestion loosened with practice. Alora asked us to perform precisely eleven minutes each day before proceeding with the second part of our meditation: *mantra.*

"Inhale slow and steady with a silent soooooooooooo ... and exhale equally slow and steady with a silent hummmmmmmmmmmmmm." Alora suggested the *so* sound naturally occurred on inhalation. Mine sounded more like huuuuhhhhh?

I found the same true for *hum*. My exhalation sounded more like ahhhhhhhhhhhh than hummmmmmmmmmmmm. Soham, *I am That*.

I imagined the sounds, which kept my focus on the breathing and my mind from wandering. My breath squeezed into my chest, unable to penetrate the bottom half of my lungs. I closed my eyes to garner control of my breath but my awareness of the group denied me the quiet solitude I enjoyed while meditating at home. Soooooooooooo. Hummmmmmmmmmmmmm.

"Practice for either eleven minutes or 108 *mala* repetitions." Alora called our attention back. I was unsure of the purpose of mala beads, but rather than speak up and sound ignorant, I decided I would google it when I returned home. Morning practice complete, we headed to the large kitchen to prepare lunch.

Each person had brought a vegetarian potluck item to share with the group. Pasta salads, couscous, taco dip with corn chips, mixed greens, even vegetarian pizzas filled the cabin's long counter and kitchen table. I added my green salad tossed with blueberries, sunflower seeds and maple dressing to the buffet. Until then, I hadn't appreciated how satisfying a vegetarian diet could be, in both nutrition and flavour. It was a treat to enjoy a meal someone else helped prepare and clean up, with adult conversation, serene surroundings and no one needing anything from me.

I sat on a large tree stump on the sunny south corner of the wood-plank deck off the sunroom, just outside the sliding door where I had placed my mat. Like a painter's palette, my plate held a small sampling of each dish to ensure everything agreed with me before I entertained a larger portion. Though my kids had dietary issues, I had none. I could pretty much eat like a goat. Too many greens or beans, however, would make for a gassy and rather embarrassing afternoon.

I listened to bits of conversation between the others but mainly we ate in silence, a silence I normally would have found awkward and tried to fill with chatter about weather, kids, the morning's activities ... anything. Sitting on the stump after over six hours of exploration, some in nature, most in my head, I happily savoured the food and the silence.

Anna and I had made a pact to use the precious time away from family commitments for ourselves, and not fill it with idle chit chat about kids, partners and day-to-day routines. It left me with little to say. Relief. I wasn't anything to anyone. I was simply there, eating, soaking up the warmth of the sun, the freshness of the air and the sound of the chickadees and sparrows chirping in the trees, dropping swiftly to the wooden planks to snatch fallen crumbs. I wasn't teaching anyone, I wasn't parenting anyone, I felt no need to do *anything*. The peace tasted as delicious as the food.

"Who made the Chinese salad?" I asked — by far my favourite.

"Oh, that was me," replied Louise. "It's such an easy dish to make. I'll give you the recipe if you like."

I liked Louise. She laughed and talked faster when she shared within the group, suggesting she was as uncomfortable in that setting as me. Her face grew red against her near shoulder-length strawberry blonde hair. A few years older perhaps, she was one of the nicest people I had met in a long time. The kind of nice that never needed guarded walls or defences to keep anyone out. A kind of nice that greeted me immediately and returned every time I commented or shared during our practice.

Hearing my description would certainly elicit that red face from her. Louise worked as a nurse in the Children's Hospital: fortunate for the kids who came into her care. Having visited the hospital on several occasions with my kids, I knew how difficult the trip could be and imagined Louise easing that burden for parents and children alike. Just like she naturally and probably unknowingly eased my discomfort in the gathering of strangers that morning.

I rinsed my dish, stacked it in the dishwasher and headed for the bathroom. The sheer curtains did little to prevent peeping in from the outdoors. Rural life. I'd forgotten.

Music limboed under the door. Jason Mraz's *I'm Yours* charmed us back to the sunroom. We would become accustomed over the year to regroup at this rhythmic cue. As with everything I had experienced so far with Alora and the group, the musical prompt provided an alternate, more elegant invitation than words.

3

THE ONLY WAY OUT IS THROUGH

"See a red ball of light at the base of your spine ... connected to a red ball of light deep in Earth's core." Soft rock gave way to primal drum. Alora closed her eyes and walked in place to the beat. We followed suit.

I maintained pace with the drumbeat. Strange, primitive chanting joined the drum and music. Alora's voice accompanied the chant and we all joined in. "*Uh ooh oh ah eye aye ee,*" we repeated over and over as the drumbeat grew louder. "*UH OOH OH AH EYE AYE EE,*" our voices rose with the drum. My steps became sloppy. Missteps, due to mis-coordination between chanting, breathing, closed eyes and trying not to move from my spot in the sunroom. I dug deeper. *Focus, Stephanie.* I found my feet again.

We held our trance-like state for what felt like an eternity, numb to time. I felt myself shifting position ever so slightly with each step, a snail's pace movement from my place of origin. Stepping, drifting, chanting, shifting.

Like a game of musical chairs, the sounds stopped suddenly, jarring me from my meditative state. I opened my eyes to see everyone spread across the entire sunroom.

Sandra faced an interior wall and appeared startled when she opened her eyes wide to discover herself nose-to-wall in a near collision.

I felt buzzed. My head hummed from the repetitive chant and my body vibrated from the continuous stepping. Not anxious or jittery, rather focused and insulated, as if the vibrations of the music, voice and movement had woven an energy cocoon around me.

Alora gathered us once more in a circle, hands extended forward and eyes closed, a running theme in the work apparently. As I stood there, I felt a cool, damp, clump placed into my hands and recognized it as clay. Once everyone held their clump, Alora instructed us to shape it, no peeking. "*Feel* the mass and *allow* it to take the form of a vessel, able to contain something."

I didn't shape it so much as I moved it from one hand to the other, pressing, feeling, pushing into it, no real design in mind. I made a concerted effort to let go of my need to control the outcome.

We each opened our eyes when we'd finished forming our vessels. I wondered, after looking at the others' creations, if I had misunderstood the instructions. My vessel looked *very* free form: a short, oval, off-centred base with thumb-grooved petals lining the edges — like something a preschooler could have made. Others' vessels looked more defined, with pleasant symmetry or clever design. I reminded myself it wasn't a competition but I wanted to repeat the exercise and make something more deliberate, something better.

So I suck at clay, big deal. It was a small deal, but that small deal caused me to pick at myself, criticize myself repeatedly. I saw the clay as something I gave form to and I didn't like the form, but it existed and I had to look at it and live with it and blame myself for not doing better. The difference between me and a preschooler? A preschooler would've been thrilled by their clay-time creation.

Alora passed around a wooden skewer and asked us to inscribe one word into the bottom of our work. I carved the word that came to me on the hill top: *FAMILY*. We took turns sharing how we felt during the molding and the significance of the word we chose. I fell deaf to the details shared by those before me, while my mind busily constructed my story.

I stated my word and my desire for harmony in the home. "I tried not to control the form of my vessel, rather allowing a more organic shape to emerge." Although the truth, it felt like I needed to explain why my sculpture sucked. I made an excuse for my poor display as if that would make me feel and appear less impotent. We set our art on a table against the far wall in the cabin's living room. Our day neared completion.

"We'll complete each gathering by stringing commitment bracelets with gemstones for each chakra." Alora spread small bags of beads on the floor in the centre of the sunroom. The bracelet represented our individual commitment to our work over the course of each forty-day period. She called it a sacred practice, to be completed in silence. *At least we get to keep our eyes open*.

She offered two options of strings for our bracelets. The first was a silk cord not easily removed without cutting or breaking the strand. The other, an elastic string which could be removed at will. I chose non-elastic after much internal debate and dialogue about how circumstances *could* arise where I *might* need to remove it. *Really, why would I need to take it off? I signed up, showed up, might as well commit to the process. After all, it's a piece of jewelry, not a tattoo.*

Each bag displayed a price sticker. We had to pay separately for our beads, which irked me since I already paid for the year. I tried not to begrudge Alora the opportunity to earn an income but my ego charged across my mind, calculator in hand, punching numbers through my brain and I rode that horse full-sweat into the barn.

Alora suggested instead of heading for the large garnets, the most decorative of the gems —and the least interesting to me — we use her pendulum[1] to ask which gem would be appropriate.

"Huh," I snorted aloud in a moment of déja vu. Weeks earlier, while making another gluten-free, dairy-free breakfast for my two small people with sensitive stomachs, I half-paid attention to the local TV morning show. A segment about Feng Shui had caught my attention; two consultants used a pendulum to determine if a space needed improvement. While holding the pendulum they asked, "Does this space need more purple?" Depending upon how the pendulum swung in their hands, the answer was either yes or no. *Wow*, I had thought, *that's really stupid*.

Alora's pendulum, a silver, cone-shaped bob clinging a silk string, lay on the floor between her and the gems. I launched myself at it. I held the pendulum over each bag of beads, asking: *Is this stone right for me?* I preferred hematite out of all the available stones. I had always loved its silvery-charcoal colour, smooth, cool surface and substantial weight. I had bought several hematite rings during my years in Banff; it was a staple in the tourist traps.

I hovered the pendulum above the smallest of the garnets, simple and round with little faceting. *Is this stone right for me?* The pendulum swung back and forth. I checked my hand and steadied it to ensure I was not directing the movement. I approached the next bag of gems, unsure of the meaning of the back and forth motion.

I continued with the medium-sized garnets. The pendulum again swung back and forth. Unable to draw any conclusions I moved onto the hematite, certain that on some subconscious level my hand would move the pendulum differently over the one I desired.

Nope. The silver decision-maker oscillated once again. Either the pendulum was hocus pocus or I didn't know how to use one. Alora had not demonstrated the technique and I wasn't about to ask for help.

I finally brought the pendulum over the large garnets. Multiple facets flicked red sunlight across the floor. *Is this stone right for me?* The pendulum traced a perfect circle, distinct from its previous pattern. Still not convinced, I repeated the entire experiment while making others wait their turn.

Same results. Only over the large garnets. *How?* My scalp tingled. I passed the pendulum to the next person, grabbed my large garnets and began to string them in silence. I recalled my reaction to the Feng Shui segment. Perhaps I should experience something before passing judgment.

I plucked a garnet from the plastic bag. *What do I want to improve in my life in relation to root chakra? Family. Okay, family.* The words flowed into each bead: support, encouragement, sleep, happy home, healthy bodies. I wanted to break the silence and visit with Anna. Our day quickly wrapped up and we hadn't visited as much as we had hoped.

Anna packed up and made her way quietly across the sunroom. She paused in the doorway, tapping at her wrist as if she wore a watch. I gave her my *What the hell was that?* look, and nodded farewell.

The gathering moved into overtime. Some collected their remaining beads and left to string at home. I knew that if I failed to finish at the cabin, it would not get done. I stayed in the quiet of the sunroom and completed my bracelet.

Alora tied it onto my wrist. Though honoured to have the teacher tie my first bracelet, it hung like a noose around my arm. It would stay until the year was over, or longer if I wished, until I felt the purpose of the inquiry into root chakra had been realized.

As awkward as much of the inquiries and exercises had felt, I experienced a deep sense of discovering something powerful and therapeutic. I thought back to my body vibrating after the walking meditation, enlivened by primal energy, then to the feeling of relief while sitting on the stump at lunch. And still further to the invocation of the prophecy and the echoing rhythm of the rattle through the valley and my mind. All events lured me into further exploration. It felt like the call to the Hero's journey that Joseph Campbell referred to, and although I wasn't ready to accept, I was intrigued enough to listen.

The experiences enticed me more than the discomfort of the process deterred me. I spent the day *feeling* more than explaining, in silence more than voice, and although that produced struggle within, something deeper convinced me there was value in the experience. The day stood on its own, pure nectar, sustaining me beyond reason, logic or form.

I RETURNED HOME and pulled into the garage. I opened the car door to yelling and loud, quick thumps of little feet scampering across the kitchen floor. Voices of television hockey commentators reverberated through the back door. I took a deep breath. The frenzy of everyday life hit me like a shock wave after my day of quiet reflection. A mixed reaction bubbled up inside me as I opened the door and set my bags, clothes and yoga mat on the floor of the back entry.

Michael and Khali came running when they heard the sound of the door close behind me.

"Mom! Mom's home, Mom's home!" Michael arrived first with a big hug. "Mom, look what I made today. It's a ship, well, not only a ship, it's a special ship. It can fly and has secret hidden lasers, like this, watch."

His twenty-one-month-old sister, Khali, beamed innocently from behind Michael as she put her arms around me and I scooped her up. I walked into the kitchen. Steve stood at the sink, finishing up the dinner dishes while he watched the hockey game.

"How was it?" he asked, his eyes on the screen.

"It was good."

I was happy to see the kids and hear about their day, but I wasn't completely there. A part of me still sat in the sun's rays on the deck, paced in place to the drum and absorbed the peace found in not being anything to anyone — but simply being.

I ran the bath and fetched pajamas from the kids' closets. I gave them a quick rinse in the tub. I wanted to head for my laptop to begin unravelling some of the day's events. I toweled off wet hair.

"Each of you grab a book, just one." I read quickly as I lay on Michael's bed, the two of them tucked under the duvet. I placed the books on the floor and kissed him goodnight. "I love you, now get some sleep."

I collected Khali in my arms and carried her off to her

bed. Another tuck under the covers, kiss on the forehead, an "I love you" and both kids were out, freeing me for research.

Steve had already taken up position in the office, busily writing software on one screen while watching the rest of the hockey game, muted, on the other. I sat down in my office chair at the long, shared desk, a couple feet away from him and googled the prophecy Alora had read earlier that day. I savoured it, recalling the lines that struck me on the hillside and dissecting lines of which I held no memory.

The prophecy had weighed powerfully when I first heard it and I felt more entranced after reading the words in the quiet of the evening. I printed a copy and placed it on my desk to read and ponder for the following thirty-nine days and beyond. I see it even now, the last line peering out at me from the stack of documents in the top bin of my filing tray, "We are the ones we've been waiting for."— The Elders, Oraibi, Arizona Hopi Nation."

4

A NEW FOUNDATION

I devoured my homework. Earth postures from our retreat practice anchored each day, complete with affirmations spoken aloud, my open journal on the floor to remember them all. I chose a mat-less practice, preferring the organic feel of dropping to the carpet in the living room, no prep or ritual required. I firmly set my postures, gaze fixed past my outstretched fingertips onto the mountains framing the skyline through the large living room window.

"My physical body is an extension of Earth. Therefore, what I do for one, I do for the other." I didn't need to drop my gaze to the page in order to recite this particular affirmation. It lingered in my memory from the previous day, when I'd chanted it in unison with the group at the lodge. "What I do for one, I do for the other." I repeated it throughout my day, probing its significance. The words tasted familiar, like a phrase from a lost page of my personal instruction manual.

As a group, we committed to read *A New Earth* by Eckhart Tolle. Root chakra homework: Chapter One. I read a few pages each day while I rode my stationary bike in our walkout basement while Khali napped and Michael was in preschool. With running and weight training off the table, the stationary bike was my refuge from a sedentary life.

I rejected the possibility of forgoing my workout. Book in hand, I leaned on the handlebars with my elbows, and stood in the pedals, tension on the fly wheel near maximum. I drove each leg downward to feel the resistance met with the strength and strain of each leg muscle. The movement strained my eyes while I focused on the words dancing on the pages before me. I declared it a challenge to my core strength and steadied my body, reducing sway and intensifying the workout. I prided myself on my level of fitness and my ability to multitask, believing both maximized my busy day as a mom.

A New Earth rang true. I did indeed feel that I was not me, not my true self. Instead, I was living how I thought I should for my age and place in life or how I perceived others expected me to live. I strove to reach the high bar I had set for myself, whether it was in parenting or career, and yet continued to push higher and higher making it impossible to ever arrive and say, "Okay, I'm here, I'm done."

What would *here* look like and what would it mean to be *done*? Wasn't that the point of life, doing and doing and doing until I did it all? What about being and being and being until I was all? I wondered what *that* looked like. Something about the paradox appealed to me. I liked the weight of it.

The homework prompted new trains of thought, many irrational. I liked how it felt to ask a question and not need to formulate the answer, instead allowing the query to hang in the air like a balloon whose string slipped through the loosely gripped fingers of a small child and floated skyward, destination unknown. I would later be freed by the insight that what I set in motion wasn't always for me to complete. The balloons I released were often for others to find. It became less about who discovered them and more about how they could be of benefit.

I earmarked my page, closed the book and dropped it to the floor. I sat, still pedalling, forcing the resistance knob to the left, eager to reduce the load on my legs and my lungs. I pushed my bangs off my forehead with the back of my hand, trying to absorb the words.

> "You do not become good by trying to be good, but by finding the goodness that is already within you, and allowing that goodness to emerge. But it can only emerge if something fundamental changes in your state of consciousness." (page 13, A New Earth)

I remembered taking an employment test thirteen years earlier, for a restaurant job in one of the hotels in Banff. Funny what stays with a person over the years. The only question I recalled was if I believed people were fundamentally good and given the opportunity would do the right thing. I answered yes, with conviction, as if it were the one question on the test I knew for certain.

I shared it, and my response, with my first husband (boyfriend at the time), an ex-police officer. He laughed and said that I was probably the only person to answer that question with a yes. He believed, given the opportunity, people would do what benefitted them, their own good, without consideration for others. I didn't agree. I felt strongly about the goodness in people.

The chapter repeatedly mentioned *a shift in consciousness*. *What does that mean? How? What would that look like?* Insights about spirituality and religion resonated deeply with me as I considered myself a spiritual person yet not a religious one, and I knew what that meant to me even if I couldn't convey it adequately in words.

People I knew either went to church and believed in God, or didn't. I believed in all sorts of things, most importantly that anything was possible and no one knew the absolute truth. I also believed my beliefs continue to change throughout my life as I taste the extensive selections of life's menu.

The ego, the running dialogue in my head, could it be responsible for my unhappiness? The question didn't float around in my mind like others. It soaked through my pores like a spring rain. It settled into my bones and flushed my veins. I felt invigorated, not by the thirty-minute cardio session, but by the possibilities. The sound of little feet on the hardwood floors above ended my allotted time for self.

I tended to meals, snacks, crafts, stories and playground time. I tidied the house and shuttled children to and from preschool. My thoughts, however, drifted constantly to the practices, the reading, the insights, the questions and the fact that I stood on a doorstep, barely through its frame, and the vast field over which I gazed, stretched ahead, enticing me to come play.

Walking meditation failed to occur daily but I managed a few. The kids happily swarmed Steve after work while I slipped out the front door. I followed the sandstone path alongside our two-story walkout. The distant mountains came into view and I emerged through the back gate: my portal from city to sacred, from responsibility to possibility, from mom and wife to Stephanie.

I breathed deeply. My shoulders unhooked from my ears with the exhalation, freedom. Freedom to get to work, homework. I visualized the red ball of light at the base of my spine connecting with the red ball of light deep in Earth's core. It focused my mind on the here and now, no room for stray thoughts replaying a recent phone conversation, a previous disagreement with Steve, a situation I handled poorly with the kids, or planning my grocery list for the following day — all regular players in the theatrical performance in my head.

It took concentration to see the two balls of light, their connection to one another, move my feet, stay on the path, breathe and occasionally close my eyes to deepen the visualization without running into a cyclist, a dog or a tree. I returned quickly, so as not to overextend my time and deprive Steve of his, and I helped get the kids to bed.

Children asleep, husband clicking away on the keyboard in the office, I closed the door to our bedroom and placed a cushion on the floor next to our bed in view of the alarm clock on the bedside table. I noted the time and closed my eyes. I wasn't a stranger to meditation. I had practiced morning and evening when pregnant with Khali, after reading Deepak Chopra's: *A Perfect Health*.

It helped, when I chose to do it: a calming and centring effect that kept me from feeling and, according to Steve, behaving frantically. I knew what he meant. Those times when twenty things ran through my head at once and I struggled to manage any of them in a calm manner.

"Someone feed the cat. I have to pack the diaper bag. Michael, get your *shoes* on! Steve, Khali needs a snack for the road." I worked myself and everyone around me into a frenzy, barking directions and rushing everyone about. Interesting how the energy of one person in the house affects everyone else. It stood to reason then, if I focused on my own happiness and health, ease would infiltrate my household.

My fear, of course, was selfishness: robbing time from the kids and Steve to focus on me. It seemed a clear choice, however: more time with frantic, disengaged Mom or less time with calm, content Mom. Quality over quantity, I chose. I preferred that the words I spoke to my family came from a place of love and support, and that those that didn't need to be spoken, weren't. I needed a break, and I began to realize it wasn't from anything or anyone other than my own internal dialogue.

I opened one eye to check the bright red digits of the alarm clock for my cue to stop breathing through one nostril, as if peeking through one eye somehow assisted me in remaining in my full meditative state. Six minutes had passed. I resumed, eyes tightly closed, determined that the next time they opened I would have made it to the finish.

Nine minutes. *Damn.* My brow furrowed. *Unclench your jaw, settle in and relax.* Finally, eleven minutes. I drew a deep breath. The air freely filled both nostrils.

Pleased with my success, I continued with mantra meditation: eleven minutes of soham, *I am that.* Again, eleven minutes felt like twenty. I periodically repeated my squinty-eyed time check to realize only a couple minutes had passed since the last check. Inhale *sooooooooooooo*, exhale *hummm-mmmmmmmmm.*

Why are you peeking at the clock? I chastised myself. *Are you concerned you'll inadvertently go over the eleven minutes? Suddenly you'll open your eyes to discover you've been lost in so hums for over an hour? Focus, Stephanie. Soooooooooo ... hummmmmmmm.*

5

ALMOND MILK, APPLES, EGGS, PENDULUM

Who knew my local organic grocery store carried pendulums? I couldn't wait to get home and try out my new purchase. Neither could Michael. *What to ask? What to ask?* I started with the obvious.

"Am I a man?" The large diamond-shaped clear crystal carved the same back and forth path I had witnessed at the yoga retreat.

"Am I a woman?" The circular pattern reappeared. I asked the pendulum all sorts of questions, as did Michael, who found success and delight in asking his age and gender.

It was my new favourite toy: the crystal consultant, a default decision maker, a source to direct my questions when I didn't want to, or couldn't, make a decision. Since kids, that was often. I deferred to my crystal regularly, giving it authority over all sorts of decisions in my life. Some decisions I made after several consultations, especially when I disliked the first answer. But if I asked the pendulum the same question too many times or too many different ways, hoping for an answer I preferred, it simply started swinging around in circles for everything as if to indicate, *If you've already decided what answer you'd like, stop wasting my time.*

It seemed silly but I felt relieved to hand over the decision-making. Having rarely slept for periods longer than two hours in over five years, I was too tired to make decisions. I second guessed most everything, doing an exhaustive "what if" scenario with every choice in my day. As if one particularly well-made decision held the key to happiness in my home.

The real issue was lodged somewhere between the lack of confidence in my decisions and the lack of trust in my inner guidance. I didn't even know what that was. From what I read, the voice of my inner guidance only emerged once I quieted the constant chatter in my mind long enough to allow it. That could take time. Most days my mind hosted a convention of thoughts, answers, guesses, judgments, critiques and scenarios. Until I could be silent and hear my inner guidance, the pendulum would provide a suitable substitute.

"Nap time, Michael. Khali's already out. How about you have a little snooze too?" Michael didn't nap anymore but his sniffles hinted at the onset of a cold, and I needed time to myself. He fought me on it. "What if you have a nap and while you're sleeping I'll boil and chill some eggs and when you wake up we will decorate Easter eggs?" Easter had just passed but the excitement lingered, enough for Michael to take the deal.

How to spend my precious free time? A quiet house, time to myself. Don't waste it. What would be the most fulfilling use of this time? I turned to the pendulum. The crystal would know. Holding my pendulum steady in one hand I asked it, "Should I do yoga?"

No. The pendulum nodded back and forth.

"Should I meditate?"

No.

"Should I write?" I felt certain that would be a yes.

No.

"Work out?"

Still no.

"Have a cup of tea and relax?!" I yelled at it.

No again.

"Take a nap?!!" By that point I was exasperated. *Stupid pendulum.*

No.

Running out of ways on how to spend my precious down time, and using up that time playing Twenty Questions with the pendulum, I paused and sat for a moment on the edge of my bed. *What to ask next? Ah ha!* "Should I boil eggs?"

The pendulum swung in circles, yes.

So I boiled eggs.

I had decided somewhere along the way that for me to benefit the most, my free time had to be only about me and not the kids or anyone else. That decision left me resentful when the kids woke early from a nap and *robbed* me of my time. Or a friend or family member called and I refused to pick up the phone because I didn't want them eating into my time. Adding the eggs to the pot of water, I discovered I didn't need to escape motherhood, escape life, to feel better about myself.

No sense of achievement required, no anxious anticipation of something or someone interrupting my important activity, I leisurely boiled eggs. I enjoyed the real gift of my down time: the tranquility I had felt sitting on the stump in the sunshine on the porch of the cabin. I placed no demands on myself. I caught a glimpse, perhaps fleeting, of an understanding of something subtle, simple, and yet empowering: life was a lot less complicated than I was making it.

Each day I returned to my mat, my particular place on the living room carpet. I slipped easily into the postures, the breath and the affirmations. I sank into the silence and the bubble of *me* time. During the forty days in root chakra, it became apparent my struggle was not with my practice. For me it wasn't about finding yoga on my mat; it was about finding yoga in the mundane act of boiling eggs.

"Give up defining yourself — to yourself or to others. You won't die. You will come to life."

~ Eckhart Tolle

PART II

SACRAL CHAKRA

SURRENDER

To feel your natural rhythm,
you have to let go of who you think you are.

6

POI PARTY

I scanned the list of unread email messages and directed my mouse click to the one marked "Water." Details of our second gathering at Sacred Forest Lodge poured from the page. Forty days had passed quickly. My routine in Earth provided a sense of stability and certainty, focusing my mind, body and breath every day. I looked forward, however, to another full day of yoga, breathing, eating, sun and life at the cabin.

"I have rented the cabin for the night before our gathering and will sleep over. Anyone who wants to join me can stay the night for a fee." Alora's email caught me by surprise.

Seriously? A good night's sleep, void of traffic noise, waking kids, middle-of-the-night train whistles and snoring husband? Sorry, Hon. I emailed Anna. She shared my excitement at the possibility of a sleepover. I called Steve at work and tested the waters. He said go. Anna and I snatched up the offer like two kids about to enjoy their first slumber party. We had no idea who else had agreed to join the sleepover and we didn't care, because we had a scheduled night off, together.

I ARRIVED at the lodge to find Anna already in the cabin, along with Alora, Kristen and Britt. I placed my bag in the red room, which I named because of the crimson linens, curtains and decorative details: découpage of red-tailed birds and red blossoms enlivened the ceiling. I unzipped a side pouch, grabbed a large, dark chocolate bar and joined the girls in the living room for a cup of tea.

I snapped the bar into pieces before opening the wrapper and set it on the table. I curled up on a corner of the couch. Anna took up the opposite corner. Alora set kindling in the large fieldstone fireplace. As the fire took hold, smoke crept out the front of the fireplace and into the room.

"I don't think the flue is open," said Britt.

Alora reached up into the mouth of the fireplace and fiddled with the damper. "I'm not sure which way it goes."

The fireplace belched out more smoke and it began to crawl along the ceiling.

"I've got it," said Britt, raising her tall, sturdy frame from her chair. She reached inside. *Thunk.* The mouth of the fire-place inhaled the escaping smoke in one deep breath.

On the table before us, Alora had spread a buffet of mystical-looking items. Colourful boxes of angel cards, tarot cards, animal cards and a bag of rune stones[1] were surrounded by mugs of tea.

I owned one deck of cards, a simple deck with Zen proverbs, a gift from Anna years ago. I drew cards from it on occasion, and enjoyed the cryptic, poetic quotes, but hadn't pulled from it in quite some time. Rune stones I'd heard of, yet we hadn't crossed paths.

I pulled from the animal deck, flipping through the

accompanying book for insight, then passed it along to Britt. Anna handed me the Goddess deck she'd just pulled from.

"If you want to work with the rune stones, hold the bag in your non-dominant hand." Alora cradled the blue velvet bag in her left hand. "Clear your mind and ask your question. Pull one stone for a simple question or you may want to pull three stones if you have a bigger issue."

I followed her instructions. Deeply coloured gemstones graced one side of the small wooden tiles. On the other side of each tile was a traditional Celtic symbol: an ornate life compass indeed.

I welcomed the company and conversation: joking about card messages with my sister cat, hearing Alora's insight and experiences with the runes and cards, and Britt's warm, no-nonsense personality. An accountant, Britt had a natural air of organization and accuracy, however, in our group, she allowed her vulnerability and softness to shine. She was a truly kind woman. Britt wore her light brown, straight hair shoulder length. Natural golden hi-lights framed her face. She and her husband lived in the hamlet with their two boys, and she regularly attended Alora's yoga classes.

I couldn't stop yawning as I drew my final cards. I desperately wanted to crawl into my comfy bed.

"Who's up for spinning?" Alora perked up.

As a personal trainer, *spinning* in my world involved stationary bikes and extended tracks of 80's remixes. I wondered where she hid the bikes. Evidently, in Alora's world, spinning involved tennis-sized plastic balls on strings looped around your fingers and propelled via wrist action in circular motions.

One poi ball on each hand contained LED lights that flashed and changed colours as they spun. I remembered watching fire spinning in Hawaii but had never experienced their training tool: the glowing poi balls. I dearly wanted to turn in and sleep but I couldn't resist the lure of the glowing balls.

Music pumping, the four of us stood in the large sunroom watching Alora skillfully demonstrate the movements. Kristen dozed on the couch. How she could sleep with such loud music was a testament to her youth.

Britt, Anna and I, strings secured to our fingers, whipped the hard plastic balls around us in circles in the dark. The neon lights reflected back at us from the wall of windows. The vibrations from the beat of the techno drum erupted from the speakers and shook my bones. My body pulsed in time with the rhythm, absorbed in an uninhibited luau: the heat, the night air, the intensity, the music, the primitive and sensual dance, until, *ouch.* I bounced one of the plastic poi balls off my head to realize they hurt, a lot.

I needed to work with the force and movement of the ball. I controlled the spinning but the ball seemed to have a mind of its own once in motion. A relaxed control held the key. Getting into the beat of the music, keeping my body fluid and using my wrist movement to guide the balls in flight so as to avoid colliding with each other or my head, allowed the kaleidoscope of colour to bounce off the windows.

The faster they spun, the more animated their pattern of light. At high speed, I merged with the rhythm of the movements and trusted my own body as well as the flight of the ball — no thinking, just flowing, moving, pulsing — a mystical display, as if the soft lights danced on their own, inviting me to join. I maintained the fluidity and pace for only a moment before my mind cut in: *I'm doing it!* And bounced yet another ball off my body.

I paused to rub my wounds and watched Alora as she

skillfully guided the lights in a wave-like pattern around her. An electric butterfly appeared in the dim light before me. Tribal, tropical, sensual, playful, powerful; I felt overtaken by the urge to surrender to the music, the movement, the night and the raw experience.

When I finally crawled into the cool sheets of the red room's queen bed, my head sunk into layers of pillows. I pulled the down duvet up around my face and basked in the stillness of the lodge and relief of knowing my ears didn't need to be on guard for calls of *Mom* in the night. My ears rang from the beating of the drums, my body vibrated from our primitive dance. I felt the distinctive essence of second chakra and fell into a glorious sleep.

7

THE MIND'S EYE DOESN'T WEAR MASCARA

I woke the next morning like a kid at Christmas. I considered lingering in my warm guest bed, but I wanted to know what gifts awaited me that day. I left my cozy down-filled cocoon and slipped out of my night shirt.

The memory of the previous night's spinning wasn't the only thing that was raw. My skin was tender. Several perfectly round bruises marred my body. *Rite of passage, I guess.*

I applied makeup and styled my hair; after all, it was a social gathering and I never presented myself to the world without a carefully crafted face: lip liner, gloss, blush, shadow, eyeliner, and, most importantly, mascara — my morning ritual since the age of fourteen. I headed to the kitchen to begin my day as usual: a cup of hot water and squeezed lemon juice. A light breakfast of oatmeal and fruit served to fuel the morning's yoga.

The members started to arrive, yoga mats and gear in hand. We greeted each other in the large kitchen while preparing tea. Alora called us to the kitchen table to meet our new "boatmate", as she referred to the newest member of our Saturday group. Lisa had switched to our Saturday community from the Sunday group, with which we'd had no interaction.

She sat at the end of the table: long, dark hair, full lips, large eyes and long eyelashes. She was wearing a tank top and an ankle-length cotton skirt — the epitome of femininity in my eyes. I guessed her age as somewhere in her early forties, slightly older than me.

Alora's reference to us as boatmates came from the Hopi prophecy that mentioned letting go of our grip on the shore and floating along with the river, looking around to see who floated with us: our community. She also called us a *sangha*, Sanskrit for assembly or community, and our year in yoga, *sahaja*, Sanskrit for natural, simple, spontaneous. I began to appreciate the eloquence of Sanskrit and how one word expressed much.

"We'll dedicate an hour or so this morning to sharing about ourselves and our stories." Alora gathered us around the large wooden kitchen table. Some, like Lisa, Anna, Louise and me, shared conservatively, as if introducing ourselves at a ladies' luncheon.

"Hi, I'm Stephanie. I'm married with two children. Anna and I have been friends for a long time, since first meeting in Banff. And I'm happy to be here."

Others shared generously: details of recent separations, difficulties with their partners, health issues and grief, complete with tissues and tears. My eyes searched for Anna's. My comfort level deteriorated from the previous lightness of tea. *Why would someone share intimate details of their life with a group of strangers?* I uncrossed and re-crossed my legs. *Am I supposed to console her? Or do I just sit here? What's the protocol?*

Why do you care what someone else shares? A voice echoed in my head. *You chose what to reveal about yourself, you had your turn, give others the same freedom.* I couldn't be vulnerable enough to share openly with strangers. Someone would surely use it against me. I viewed the emotional displays as weakness yet coveted the freedom the women felt to express so purely and completely. Still, my mind despised the victim, denying it in myself.

Each time a judgment arose about a member of the group, I saw its connection back to me, like looking in a mirror. My mind thought the issues belonged to the other, yet that "other" drew out my own issues. I looked at Jill and listened to her story, her sobbing. I saw myself. At that moment I saw fear, vulnerability and the need to cover it up.

The mirror reflected the negative in me. Then I remembered my earlier thoughts about Lisa and her raw beauty; perhaps the mirror also reflected the beauty in me. Maybe it reflected the beauty that I failed to acknowledge in myself. Perhaps the natural femininity I appreciated in Lisa also existed unrecognized in me.

With a dozen women sharing around the table, tea flowing as freely as the tears and stories, time passed quickly; nearly two hours had elapsed. We rinsed our mugs in the sink and moved to the sunroom to begin second chakra practice.

We sat on our mats while Alora discussed the new focus of our forty-day practice: second chakra, sacral chakra, *svadhisthana*, Sanskrit for *one's own place*. The chakra is associated with water, flow and movement. Second chakra corresponds to the colour orange and it governs the sexual organs, fertility, birth, rebirth, renewal and change.

"Second chakra also governs emotions," said Alora, "particularly guilt."

Sacral chakra fosters creative expressions of all kinds including art, dance, fashion, jewelry, play and sexuality. Second chakra involves finding the sweetness in life, our inner child and inner goddess.

Alora talked about our place in the tribe. Second chakra houses our relationships, our communities, our place within communities, and how we relate to others in our lives. The second chakra mantra of *let go, let flow,* expresses the qualities of water and moving easily with the current and not against it. It encourages fluidity in life, in movement, in thinking, in feeling and in relationships, allowing one to loosen their firm grip and float effortlessly along the stream of life.

As I sat on my mat listening to her words, I thought about water in all its forms. Water holds the power of persistence and perseverance. A constant stream eventually wears away plants, earth and even rock. A single drop focused continuously and patiently over time, carves its mark in the place it lands. A torrential downpour or a tidal wave holds the potential of destruction and complete transformation of the landscape. A calm pool, the original mirror, reflects all that surrounds it, perfectly and peacefully. One ripple in that pond and images become distorted.

Alora placed large sections of canvas on top of our mats, nearly covering the entire surface. In our email list of requirements, she had listed crayons or felts, of which I had many. I had raided Michael and Khali's stash. We laid an assortment of art supplies on the floor next to our mats while Alora described and then demonstrated a flowing yoga asana practice dedicated to water.

We followed her lead. I allowed my body to move organically, naturally in the poses, assimilating the qualities of water: fluid, easy, continuous. The movements departed strongly from that of our Earth chakra practice, where I felt form, stability, solidity, and structure. I left my technically executed and firmly planted form of downward dog for a yummy dog, lapping up the waves of movement as my elbows bent, shoulders rolled and spine undulated. Well, gently undulated in my case. With each curving of my back, I tested the waters of my spine. *Careful.* I passed the movement onto my hips which, out of the blue, had locked up just days before our gathering. I rocked side to side, knees bending and heels lifting, planting, lifting, planting. Fluidity required effort at first — concentration to get the body to assume a natural rhythm. After a few moments, the rhythm washed away the mind and propelled the movement.

"Close your eyes," Alora cooed. "Notice anything flowing into your mind — ideas, judgments, thoughts — just notice as these same items flow out."

I allowed the movement of my mind to join my body.

"Renewal, release, rejuvenation," Alora suggested. "Any tension dissolving. Anything rigid, ideas or body, softening."

Each exhalation found within it a long, slow, audible sigh.

"Aaaaaahhhhhhhh," sighed Alora, "Letting go, letting flow."

"Aaaaaahhhhhhhh," the group echoed.

"Write down whatever wants to express itself through your flowing practice ... images, words, thoughts or colours that surface while you move."

I imagined throwing down a couple drawings for show. I hadn't experienced the *visions* and *inner guidance* others in the group occasionally referred to. I also hadn't done much in the way of art since my teens, with the exception of preschool-style stickmen and smiley-faced suns drawn in crayon at the kitchen table with Michael and Khali.

As my body continued to expand and move in all directions throughout the yummy dog and cat poses, I noticed Yvonne reach for her crayons. Alluring and soft-spoken Yvonne walked with grace and dressed with seductive, creative flair. Her black cotton leggings revealed the flesh of her thighs beneath patterned lace. A flowing top draped over her pants as softly as her dark blonde, wavy hair draped over her face. I wondered at what point in my practice I needed to add a few stick men to my canvas.

I closed my eyes, returning to the wave of my breath and body. My hips rocked side to side and my head dropped toward the mat in surrender to the waves rolling up my spine. *Let go.* I encouraged my fear of pain to release its grip on my mind and muscles. Images emerged from nowhere. A large open eye, complete with long lashes, appeared in my *mind's eye.* A dolphin followed. Grey-blue iridescent skin sparkled as it crested the surface of the water. I forced my eyes open, wide in disbelief. I saw them, yet I didn't see them, not with my eyes anyway. I knew them, detailed in design yet vague in purpose, not a memory.

I dropped to my knees and tried to replicate the images on my canvas, making two attempts at the curve of the dolphin's back. I still saw it clearly in my mind but my hands couldn't reproduce the shape. I drew quickly, afraid the visions would fade as fast as they appeared.

I returned to the rhythm of the waves, surprised by how easily I slipped back into the flow. More visions surfaced, cresting the waters of my practice. I continued to draw, colour and record the spontaneous display in my head, swept away in the process.

There was more happening than yoga: a surreal experience, like an enchanting dream full of life and magic, yet I was a participant in this dream, recording its details and exploring its meaning as I explored movement in my body. It was as if, as I moved, ideas and images dislodged from my joints, memories broke free of my bones — released from their bodily cage, long held hostage. The sacred rhythmic union of body and breath aroused creativity.

I recorded the bizarre details and inhabitants of this strange territory for later analysis. As long as they continued to dance before me, I continued to capture them on canvas. Although the visions opened up to me, my artistic talent remained confined.

I surveyed my canvas, post-practice, exhausted from the continual movement and capturing of visions. Those detailed images, so intriguing in my mind's eye, still resembled stick figures and smiley-faced suns. Among the many pictures and symbols that appeared to me, my curiosity followed one recurring image. I approached Alora to ask what the symbol might mean.

An eye, just one, repeated on my canvas, large, open and indigo: an impressive and compelling icon.

"Oh, how wonderful! Yes." According to Alora, both the eye and colour held significance. "The eye symbolizes inner vision, higher knowledge and awakening. Indigo is sixth chakra, third eye, intuition."

I would have continued disbelieving in my ability to have a glimpse into the unknown, perhaps into myself, had I not experienced it. The word *awakening* became the under-current of my exploration. *What is waking up in me?*

I returned to my mat and canvas, admiring my work and excitedly awaiting a turn to share my experience with the group. Yvonne held up her artwork for everyone to see. Envy coloured my vision. Her entire canvas erupted with imagery, right to the frayed edges of the fabric. Pastels imparted texture to an impressive tree, which popped off the canvas as if it were alive. Her images pulsed with rich colour.

My canvas paled in comparison: the rough sketches of eyes, faint penciled outlines of dorsal fins — drawn and redrawn — devoid of depth, of texture, sparse against the vast, beige background of the canvas. *Whatever. Something else I suck at.* My experience overpowered my ineptitude, for neither the large eye on my canvas, nor the one in my mind, appeared to require additional flare. *I* may have needed to present my face perfectly to the world, but after witnessing the workings of my mind's eye, I delighted in the simple, reflective display: no mascara required.

8

THE VIBRATION OF CHEESE

I walked into the kitchen. Britt was balancing the fridge door with her hip as she pulled the components of her potluck lunch from the shelves. She held a wrapped cheese in her hand and I peered at the label.

"I love gouda," I spouted.

"Howda," Britt corrected me in a thick Dutch accent and firm voice, so deep that it vibrated the word and drove her point home. Her warm smile and eyes contradicted her commanding stature and tone. She was the combination of strength and warmth. I still hear her every time I buy my favourite cheese and I mimic "howda." The sound begins deep in my diaphragm, propelled upwards by my core, over the back of my tongue, and forcefully escapes my throat — a whole-body experience just for cheese.

With lunch cleared away, we headed outside to meet our guest facilitator. A young girl, perhaps in her early twenties, with long, straight, mousy-brown hair stood waiting. A casual, fitted, cotton tank top and flowing skirt with thick bands of colour draped to mid-calf, and embellished her tall, thin frame. She held a large, rainbow hula hoop in one hand and an assortment of decorative scarves in the other. She handed each of us a scarf to tie around our waists. Interesting how the simple addition of a silky, flowing scarf instantly made me feel more feminine.

Next came the hoops, not ordinary hoops, but handmade. Filled with water and wrapped in bright fabric, they dually represented second chakra. We removed our shoes and spread out along the lawn beside the horse pasture, scarves draping from our midsections, hoops poised in place above our hips, toes feeling the grass and ... occasionally some dried horse droppings.

Believing we all remembered the technique, we started frantically whipping our bodies around and looked more like we were overtaken with seizures than playing a childhood game. Nothing graceful about it. Hoops fell to the ground or collided with one another. Bodies contorted in awkward movements in desperate attempts to keep the props airborne. Evidently, we remembered little.

Our facilitator politely asked us all to stop, though her tone indicated annoyance. She began to spin the hoop in her hands. She seduced the circle rhythmically and methodically from hands stretched above her head, down over her shoulders, around her waist, from leg to leg, back up over her shoulders and off above her head: elegant, gentle, sensual, lovely and effortless. She danced with the hoop as her partner.

She then broke down the movements, helping us to find the slow, even rhythm of the hoop and our hips. I felt the weight of the hoop and the plastic uncomfortably collide with my hip bones on each forced rotation. With time, I felt the natural circular flow of my hips supporting the hoop while the momentum of its inner fluid kept it afloat.

I stepped out with one leg, then the other, moving my

body in circles. My arms and hands expressed the dance further as I reached above my head, feeling the rhythm. Playful and feminine, free and creative, and exhausting. After nearly two hours of communing with the hoops, I was happy to return my borrowed scarf, hand in my hoop and sit on the grass for a drink of water. My hips continued to pulse as if they still propelled the hoop.

We remained outside for the final facilitator of second chakra activities. Alora asked us to take time in silence with the land: to walk and collect small twigs and leave a traditional offering of sugar or tobacco in their place. My bag of sugar in hand, since I didn't stock tobacco in my pantry, I tiptoed around the property in imposed silence, trying to avoid eye contact with others for fear of breaking some rule.

I attempted to walk where no one else was walking. Alora had instructed us to stay within a certain area. That made it difficult to not cross silent paths with another. I left common ground and stepped up onto the white, wooden fence boards of the horse pasture. I side-stepped along, following the fence and wondering how many twigs to gather, running out of sugar.

I caught the attention of a few furry, four-legged residents. I leaned over, extending my hand to lure the horses. They obliged and sauntered over, as several other twig gatherers joined me on the fence to scratch furry chins and velvety soft noses.

Steve and I had put Michael into soccer, as parents do when kids express an interest. Perhaps it was more of our interest expressed than his. Michael's attention rarely stayed with the play and games often ended in him leading his fellow teammates off the field to pick dandelions. As I looked along the fence at the long line of twig gatherers, it occurred to me either Michael took after his mother or I had the attention span of a five-year-old.

Sure, I'd jumped from one job to the next, one career to the next, occasionally one boyfriend to the next in my earlier years, but what's wrong with picking dandelions? If we're so focused on the task at hand, is it possible we're missing the beauty that surrounds us? And if we're lost in the beauty that surrounds us, do we miss the task at hand? I don't have the answers.

Alora called us together and we followed her to a clearing where a woman stood opposite a fire, her hair as vibrant, orange and wild as the fire itself.

"This is my friend, Karen," Alora said. "She's a trained Shaman."

I'm not sure which mesmerized me more: the ravenous fire in front of me or her hair. Karen talked briefly about her travels to Peru and about the Incan fire ceremony in which we were about to participate. It was my first official fire ceremony — if you don't include the time Mom left a pan of oil on the stove and it caught fire, Dad swinging the kitchen floor mat over it in an attempt to extinguish it, and me running out the front door. Quite frankly, I held a hefty fear of fire.

That fear had made my first post-secondary experience a tricky one since Bunsen burners were a tool of the trade in Chemical Technology. I had managed to control my fear enough to get through my experiments, often asking my lab partner to fire up my burner. Always happy when it was time to extinguish the flame, one day I turned off the burner, unscrewed the clamp that held the metal o-ring where my beaker had perched, and headed to the sink to rinse my glassware. I returned to my station, forgetting the metal ring had just been heated to over one thousand degrees Celsius, and picked it up to put it away. It was an interesting visit to the nurse's office. On campus, the E.M.T. students practiced their skills on wounded students. I came out of the office looking like Minnie Mouse with my enormous white hand of gauze. I did not consider fire my friend.

Karen lifted her arm from beneath her thick, colourful woolen poncho and revealed a rattle. She held it out in front of her and began the custom of creating sacred space. We turned toward each direction with her as she shook the rattle and spoke to the spirits. Although the purpose and intent was similar to Lil's invocation atop Two Pine during our first chakra retreat, Karen's words differed since they stemmed from the Incan tradition rather than the Hopi. I followed along. One word resonated. It echoed through my head in a whisper, *Pachamama*.

Karen then demonstrated the many layers involved in the fire ceremony. She invited us to begin as she sang, chanting in an unfamiliar language. We approached the fire one by one while the rest chanted with Karen and held space: a kind of energetic support allowing the person at the fire to be open, vulnerable and present with their experience. Kneeling at the blaze, we blew our intentions or prayers into the twigs we'd gathered, and then placed them one at a time into the flames.

Using the action of our hands, we unwound the energy of our lower chakras, releasing into the fire that which no longer served us: beliefs, behaviours, circumstances. We filled this newly created space with the light and energy of the fire of transformation by symbolically taking the fire with our hands into our chakras, winding them back up. We repeated this process with the upper chakras.

What the hell? What an awkward exercise. Should I go up first or would that look too eager? Do I kneel close to the fire or away? How many offerings should I give to the fire? Am I supposed to move my hands clockwise to release what I no longer want and counter clockwise to bring in the light of the fire? Or counter clockwise to release and clockwise to bring in? When I hold space for the others should I put my hands out? Other people are. Should I follow or be cool and do my own thing?

I held my ground and focused on the chanting and mastery of the words, singing loudly with Karen, keeping the energy and momentum of the practice high as it took each person what seemed like forever with the fire — a lot of chanting. Singing made me feel purposeful, and it provided a way to channel my nerves. I suddenly wished I was back around the kitchen table with the awkward emotional outpouring.

I let my voice rise and join with Karen's as the voices of the others dulled and faded with the length of the ceremony. The chant gifted me an almost mind-numbing rhythm in its repetition, vibrating my lips and my entire body. The meaning of the words unknown to me, their sound rattled my bones, my whole body hummed.

What if there is actually something to this? What if I stumbled upon something powerful? I watched the person at the fire and decided to go next. The chant had shifted something in me and, with it, my thoughts. The repetitive vibration somehow coaxed possibility from discomfort. The person at the fire stood. I dropped my hands and voice, and headed to the hearth. I kneeled. With my sticks in my lap, I took a long, slow inhale, closed my eyes and exhaled to steady myself.

I let go of which direction to wind my hands. I focused instead on blowing my prayers into the twigs. I prayed for a healthy family; a happy family; a safe family; for Mom and

Dad; for Steve and me; for Michael and Khali. I set my twigs in the fire, lost in time, kneeling on the ground.

Once back in the circle with the others, I felt my time at the fire was too brief. I wanted to return, take my time with the experience and sit with the fire. I vibrated from head to toe from the chant I sustained so long with Karen. Its signature engraved on my body like the rhythm of the water-filled hoop on my hips, the oceanic movements of the morning's yoga practice, and even the vibration of Britt's *howda*. My body hummed with the frequencies of song, yoga, play and cheese.

9

A COSMIC WHODUNNIT

I stood alone, away from the fire and the group. A sudden forceful wind charged me head-on. Every hair on the back of my neck stood like quills on a porcupine. The gale appeared from nowhere. I had come to recognize the tingling as a type of affirmation: as if my body prompted me to pay attention to whatever experience or thought engaged me at that moment. This was by far the most intense wave I'd felt.

I looked around at the trees, the sky, the field, fully expecting to see someone there. It was as if someone *was* there and I knew it, felt it, but couldn't see them. As if someone arrived on that strong gale and stood there with me, speaking to me, and part of me heard them. But the other part of me, the part that worked out, the me that cooked, cleaned, tucked the kids into bed, watched TV and drank tea with friends — that part of me couldn't hear.

I stood, frozen, looking at someone, but no one was there. I felt them. *Who? How do you know it's a "them"?*

They surrounded me. The quality of the air changed: dense and full. Spirits, ancestors, energy? I didn't know details. I simply knew something communicated with me. As if Nature, herself, called to me; yet the wind wasn't soft and gentle, but forceful and powerful like an ancient energy: Earth's council.

Could it be the trees, standing witness to our ceremony? I felt that whatever it was knew of my awareness, as if they'd chosen to reveal themselves to me at that moment, alone and removed from the chatter of the group. I started a silent conversation with the unknown.

I know you know me but I can't see you.

Had I opened a door to heightened awareness, of connection and communication in this sacred space of nature, community and ceremony?

Trees, breeze, echoes of myself? Who are you?

As a child I thought we must be ignorant to think we were the only intelligent life. As a young girl, my mind was riddled with possibilities. Why did people not believe in clairvoyance or claircognizance: the ability to know something without knowing how you know it? I experienced the phenomenon as a kid in math class. I would know the answer but when the teacher asked me to show my work, I had no idea how I knew the answer. I just knew. Wouldn't that be a lot less exhausting, not having to show your work?

As a child I wrote poetry. It wasn't something I had set out to do; it seemed to find me in my sleep. I kept pen and paper by my bed and woke in the night to scribble down words in the dark then drift back to sleep to complete the work in the morning light.

I never questioned the origin of the words. Did they slip from my psyche while I surrendered to slumber? Were they adrift on a dream or wafting in the ether of astral travel? At Nan's encouragement, I had submitted one of those poems to the city fair and won fourteen dollars. I wish I could recall the words, the cadence, the subject, the message. What cosmic creativity did I glean as a child in the night?

Then again, memory is a fickle friend. I remembered myself an adept poet, yet in my early forties Mom found those treasures from elementary school that she'd kept. Among them: a collection of seasonal holiday poems. And they *stunk*.

Nan had bought me a set of Agatha Christie novels one Christmas: one of my most cherished presents. I was always intent on solving the crime before the detective: to beat the great Hercule Poirot to the reveal of whodunnit. As I remember, it didn't happen often, if at all; Christie's books were so cleverly crafted. As a bright and confident twelve-year-old, I felt certain I would solve the next one.

After the fire ceremony, I remembered what I contemplated so relentlessly as a child. There was something greater around me, and the possibility to connect with the unknown and unseen proved intensely compelling. The reclaimed curiosity of childhood reinvigorated my spirit. The race resumed. I had cracked the stiff binding on an old mystery and was certain, this time, I would beat Monsieur Poirot to the reveal.

10

BREAKING BREAD, AND BARRIERS, WITH MY SON

I opened the email entitled *Breaking Bread for Women.* It was an invitation to a potluck lunch from Alora. I first heard of the organization that initiated the charity potluck gatherings, Canadian Women for Women in Afghanistan, from my aunt Joyce. The format involved hosting a potluck and inviting nine guests. Each person contributed seventy-five dollars to the cause as well as a dish for the meal. Guests enjoyed a bountiful feast with family and friends and the charity received seven hundred and fifty dollars, the cost of one teacher's annual salary in Afghanistan.

What a great opportunity to give to others and introduce Michael to giving as well. I checked my calendar to find the date coincided with my scheduled day as the designated volunteer at Michael's preschool, as well as the Mothers-Day tea. We would need to head straight from the tea to the potluck, fruit salad in hand.

I replied to the email, intent on attending. Second-guessing set in the following day. *Why am I overextending myself and dragging Michael along on the thirty-minute drive?* It would be easier to simply stay home.

I don't know which was greater: my guilt over ditching twenty-three-month-old Khali with Steve — who already took the morning off work to cover my volunteer shift — or my fear over a possible public outburst if Michael pulled a tantrum, which would result in a test of my parenting skills, followed by more guilt over bringing a five-year-old to a charity event.

Born with reflux, Michael's regulated diet of mainly gluten-free and dairy-free foods helped him sleep at night with minimal discomfort or additional intervention; no more raising the head of the bed or wedging layers of pillows beneath his head, and no more inflammation, upset tummy or mouth breathing at night. Quite frankly, the potluck buffet put me in the middle of a guilt sandwich: the guilt over limiting his choices at the lunch and the guilt of allowing him free reign, resulting in subsequent discomfort and sacrificing his, my and potentially the entire household's sleep. I swam in guilt and I hadn't even gotten to the event. Did I mention guilt lives in second chakra?

I wanted to go. I wanted to spend time with Michael. Since Khali's birth, he and I spent little time together, just the two of us. The cause interested me and I felt community should include children, without parents worried about inappropriate behaviour. I thought people needed to loosen up, only, I didn't realize *people* meant me.

I pulled up the email invitation again. Lunch was at twelve, followed by a brief presentation by one of the organizers. I decided to attend the lunch and bolt directly afterward so as not to disturb the presentation or risk an outburst, should Michael not wish to sit through the event. It seemed a long way to go for a short lunch. *Sigh*. I looked forward to getting out of the house, however, sitting at a table enjoying a lunch I didn't have to prepare — save the fruit salad —and experiencing a change of scenery dressed in my big-girl clothes.

We entered the building and I surveyed the crowd. The gathering of over thirty-five women of all ages supporting the cause in their community, was inspiring. Lively chatter among small groups of ladies indicated most of them were familiar with one another. Other than Alora, I knew no one. She stood by the front door in deep conversation with another woman. None of my boatmates made it to the event.

Tables played host to bags, jackets and purses, and I wasn't sure where to sit. We made our way to the side of the community centre where the bazaar was. Three tables displayed exotic necklaces, rings, bracelets and earrings made with gemstones, as well as pencil cases, scarves and bags in rich fabrics. To my surprise, Michael enjoyed perusing the items as much as I, pointing out which necklaces he thought I might like. He chose a pencil case. I took his advice and claimed a hand-carved, jade bead, multi-strand necklace. We walked toward the arrangement of lunch tables, happy with our purchases, all for a good cause, of course.

Still no place to sit. Maybe we shouldn't have come. My face flushed as I stood there with Michael, the only child in the room. Standing near the buffet, his eyes widened as he inched toward the assortment of dishes. I habitually surveyed the items, assessing the few he could tolerate.

"Come, sit here with us girls," An older woman called to us from her table of friends. It was a welcome offer. I didn't have to abandon ship after all.

We left our items and coats at the table and made our way to the buffet. Michael licked his lips in pure anticipatory delight, his eyes as big as saucers; I suddenly let go of the need to act as monitor. My neck muscles relaxed; ease found my brow. "You can choose whatever you like. Enjoy." Saying those words felt like a gift for the both of us.

I watched as he deliberately made each selection, carefully spooning items onto his plate like they were diamonds, taking great care not to drop one. Baked beans, cold meats, cheese and grapes, his choices were thoughtful. It felt good to relax and let go of the negative energy surrounding him and food. I enjoyed watching him make his choices almost as much as he enjoyed making them. He particularly enjoyed the butter tart and inhaled it with enthusiasm.

"You sure seem to like your food, young man." The ladies at our table engaged Michael, asking him questions about school. They seemed delighted to have his young energy at the table.

"Can I have another butter tart, Mom?"

"Of course," I said, "last one."

As he returned to the table, the woman hosting the event stood to address the group and introduce the cofounder of the organization. My window of escape had closed.

As the cofounder shared the story of the organization, Michael devoured his second butter tart. Her experiences, vision and celebration of the beautiful, bright-eyed Afghanistan girls — newly empowered with the gift of books and literacy — were equally compelling and evocative. My attention strayed only briefly from her thirty-minute presentation when Michael finished his butter tart and I assured him we would soon leave.

I connected for a moment with Alora on our way out but it was the connections I experienced with the women at our table, feeling a part of the community as the story of other communities of women unfolded before me, that left me with the feeling of inclusion.

The best part was the time with Michael. There was no over-mothering or worrying if he would act *appropriately,* needing to bolt early from the building if things weren't going well. I enjoyed hanging out with him, without the parental anxiety I had anticipated, rather, *obsessed* over.

I realized I hadn't transitioned from toddler to child with Michael. Khali was born when he was three and I returned to the persona of *mother of an infant,* not acknowledging Michael's own shift from rambunctious toddler to curious child. The event felt like a milestone in our relationship: honouring our short journey together so far, and welcoming a new leg of that journey.

I backed the car out of the parking lot and pointed it back down the highway for the return drive home. In the rearview mirror, I watched Michael's eyelids grow heavy with long blinks. I thought about the event. I valued giving and the sense of community attached, groups of women coming together to make a difference. In staying at home with my young children, independent as I was, I missed the connection of community. At some point in my life as a parent, independence had become separation.

To this day, I can't remember if we endured a food-induced sleepless night or not. Funny, that. I only remember it as a cherished time and lovely lunch with Michael.

LETTING FLOW

I hated public pools. The thought of putting my body, let alone my face, in a chemically-treated vat of other people's bath water disgusted me. I loved the pool as a kid. I think I started to dislike it when my hair and makeup became more important than my fun.

Aunt Joyce had recommended yoga and swimming as my options for exercise, ones that posed little risk of further deterioration of my spine. Khali had started swim lessons and I decided to take the plunge into second chakra and place her in an un-parented class while I swam laps in the large pool next to her. While most parents sat, coffee in hand, watching their kids cannonball off the ledge of the kiddy pool, I planned to breaststroke my way back and forth through the bobber-lined lanes of the lap pool, careful not to put my face in the water.

I purchased a new one-piece bathing suit, possibly my first serious swim uniform for serious business. Normally, I would have opted for a stylish bikini. I stood on the edge of the lap pool, reading the instructions on the board for lane swimming. Everyone else seemed to know the drill. I watched the swim caps and goggles emerge from the water in regular intervals like a pod of dolphins.

One of the bobbing heads approached me and surfaced, as if he could tell I was a rookie to the rules of the lanes. In the water everyone looked the same, save for speed. Once emerged, I realized the fellow engaging me was at least seventy. He broke the surface tension and welcomed me by sharing the etiquette of the lap pool.

Once I understood the lay of the landless, I thanked him and gingerly lowered myself into the water, an inch at a time, allowing each section of my body to acclimate to the cold. I waited for the proper spacing to keep a safe distance from the dolphins in the slow lane. I pushed off the wall. My body found the familiar flow of the breaststroke it knew as a kid.

I aimed my focus at second chakra: water and fluidity. I watched my commitment bracelets in the ripples of my outstretched arms. The orange of second chakra carnelian and the deep reddish brown of first chakra garnet, glistened like ancient treasures in blue water.

I invited the water into my body, replenishing and revitalizing each cell, as if the water rehydrated every molecule in me. I welcomed water into the damaged discs of my once youthful and healthy spine. I envisioned the discs drinking up the water and returning to their nourished state.

I surrendered to the water, allowing it to support me and help me glide effortlessly through it. It wasn't the usual struggle or strain of exercise or swimming, but a letting go and letting flow of myself and my need to control. I floated with the water and remembered another time I had allowed myself to surrender.

At some point during my recovery years earlier, in the thirty-three days that I was bed-ridden, I had relinquished control. With no other choice, no physical option to push through the injury as with previous injuries, I let go of everything. Nearly everything. I never entertained the possibility of not recovering; I believed completely in my eventual healing.

The rest — my job, fear of loss of ground or clients, any need to look after anyone, watch the clock, attain something, achieve something, go anywhere or do anything — I let go. No amount of strain, force or control was going to heal me. My body, through my injury, had made certain that surrender remained my only option; voluntary movement was near impossible.

I gave in to the injury, to my bed and the stoppage of time. Fascinating thing, that, when injured, when unable to join in the regular routine of life's pace, time holds no power. I could see how, with a prolonged illness, however, time might work in the opposite direction and days could begin to feel endless.

Much constriction came from the struggle against time: *Not enough hours in the day; I'm late; I'm behind schedule; they've got too much time on their hands; I'm pressed for time; we're racing against the clock; if I can find the time; it's a waste of time; it's time to move out; it's time to grow up; it's time to move on; it's time to get to work; it's time ...* The number of common phrases referencing time suggested I wasn't alone in the time tug-o-war. Or, perhaps, it was those same phrases that conditioned my relationship with time.

It seemed time and fluidity were opposite sides of the same coin. They existed together, yet at odds. I wondered why time held a grasp on me, why I gave it so much power and why, once forced to relinquish its pull, I felt immense peace. I felt flow.

Unable to understand it at the time of my injury, nor appreciate the significance of flow, I simply savoured the moments in bed. I cherished the sun's light playing off the neighbour's windows behind our home, illuminating my room. The spring breeze danced across my face through the window, delivering the fresh scent of warming earth under melting snow. Unable to rush about, my senses alerted me to simpler pleasures. Everything felt more alive. It reminded me of life on the farm. Maybe one of the reasons we have such vivid memories of our childhood is because children aren't hostage to time. They live in the rich tones of the moment.

Steve had set up the TV at the foot of the bed during my recovery and I watched hours of *Home Makeover* and *The Food Network*, something I thought a waste of time before my injury. Laid up in bed it appeared as though I suddenly had all the time in the world. No one needed me. I couldn't do anything for anyone anyway. In fact, for the first time in a very long time, *I* needed someone.

Anna came by with my favourite venti beverage and we lay on the bed watching *Thelma and Louise,* sipping our over-sized drinks. Heaven. Steve's best friend and his wife stopped by with a mushroom and asparagus casserole in hand. I was being looked after, something I hadn't allowed anyone to do in a long time.

As I glided through the water in the pool, the story of my back emerged through second chakra. The position of the injury along my spine, the lack of flow in my life, and the emotions tied up in my inability to be vulnerable, all spilled out into the water around me. It was time to remove the armour I had spent years constructing. If I didn't, I would eventually sink. I just didn't know how to take it off without feeling raw and exposed.

I surrendered to the water and allowed it to carry me. I felt renewed in the pool and excited to return again each week. Khali learned to swim, and I learned to flow.

12

LETTING GO

I parked my car in the lot of the women's health centre. I rushed inside, up three flights of stairs and into the classroom. I set down my notepad, pen and water bottle on the table and took my seat left of Aunt Joyce, who was chatting with her friend sitting to her right. It was the last class in a series of four weekly seminars we attended together. The classes introduced *Ayurveda*[1], the *doshas*, yoga and breath as practices for balancing health.

Our soft-spoken facilitator started off the class with chair yoga. She then led us in a breathing exercise. I followed her lead, taking a deep breath and holding it as long as I could, not allowing the exhalation.

"Hold it, hold it," she gently encouraged the group.

I strained. *Is this safe?*

"And let it go."

I was never so relieved to release a breath.

"Now exhale completely and keep the air out as long as possible."

My head began to spin. *Am I going to pass out?* I forced my body to comply, not entertaining the thought of aban-

doning control of the breath in order to restore comfort to
my body.

"Aaaaaaaand inhale."

Thank God. I took a long, slow drink of air. I swallowed,
finishing with an audible sigh of satisfaction as if I'd just
downed a bottle of water after a workout.

"The purpose of this exercise is to demonstrate how
hard it is to keep something out that needs to come in, and
to keep something in that needs to be let go."

Her words, "let go" echoed those of Alora's and the
essence of the forty-day theme. A simple exercise, controlling my breath, made me realize perhaps I tried to control a
whole lot more in my health, my family and my life, and
quite possibly with the same panicky, frantic, and dizzying
results.

Throughout the seminars, I had learned about the
issues of other attendees. Some of the women were working
through physical issues and injuries — cancer, head trauma
and disability — while others dealt with emotional issues.
Toward the end of class, one woman shared about the aban-
donment by her father and how she had come to accept it,
forgiven him and understood the motivating circumstances.
I couldn't help but wonder if she'd really come to terms with
it. *If you are healed, why do you still identify with it? Why are
you still acting like a victim? Why are you still talking about it?*

I remembered the morning of sharing around the cabin
kitchen table, another group of women, mainly strangers,
wielding intimate details of their lives. *What is it with groups
of women and emotional outpouring? I signed up to learn about
Ayurveda, not hear about your problems.* A cold thought, yet
an honest account of my thinking at the time.

The truth about how I related to women through
competitive practices rather than supportive ones, bounced

off the old structures trying to hold their ground in my mind. Independent, I believed I conquered hurdles on my own. I'd separated myself as a young woman, a business woman, a new parent — in each stage, determined to handle life myself; certain vulnerability would mean surrendering to another. And I had viewed surrender as the greatest weakness of all.

As the woman shared further details of her father leaving, I began to feel sad for her: a beautiful middle-aged woman, caught up in the misery, anger, hurt, grief, and whatever other feelings she may have experienced, for most of her life. What a waste — the event consumed and drained her life and energy.

Why do we hold onto our stories so tight? How can we release them like we released the breath after the long-held inhale? Maybe the same forum that prompted the emotional outpourings also provided the potential to release and heal. Perhaps gatherings of women in supported community provided the vehicle to let go, let emotions flow, and allow healing to begin. Maybe all we needed was to exhale. Together.

13

THE RHYTHM OF YOGA

I drew the back of my tongue toward my throat. Alora had prescribed wave breathing, or *Ujiya* breath, to accompany our second chakra asana practice. The wave-like sound created during the slow, smooth flow of breath through an intentionally constricted opening of the throat, mimicked the ocean. I struggled to maintain the breath as I moved through the postures.

I struggled with much of my second chakra routine. Alora had stated the importance of not leaving Earth practice behind, instead building on it. I think I got washed away in the wave of second chakra. The structure of root chakra practice disappeared and my *svadhistana* practices spilled out all over my day with no form or direction. Most days the tide came in before I had a chance to get to my asana practice.

A witching hour plagued our home. Between four in the afternoon and shortly after my husband returned from work, somewhere around five-thirty, people in my home got cranky, little people and big. The kids morphed into *hangry* monkeys in need of an outlet for their excess energy while I required a means to find quiet after a day of noise, meals, cleanup and running around for groceries or preschool commutes.

Michael and Khali vied for my attention and played tug-o-war with my least nerve. I climbed upstairs to the bonus room, wading through an ocean of wooden alphabet blocks, stuffed animals, cups, plates and pots from the play kitchen, and flipped on the stereo. I returned downstairs, where I turned up the volume to the living room speakers.

A beat kicked in and two little people ran to the cream carpet: my living room yoga mat now a dance floor. Faces beamed as small bodies flailed to the rhythm. I jumped on the dance floor and executed my best funky chicken, flapping my wings and strutting across the carpet. Michael took centre stage atop the brown leather storage chest and gave a star performance. Khali happily bobbed up and down, taking great delight in her brother's crazy moves. My dance steps, more conservative and choreographed than the kids, led me around the living room, checking my form in front of the large mirror above the couch.

We grooved to several songs, the kids continuing on the dance floor while I heel-toed it into the kitchen in my signature move. I wiggled and sang as I chopped carrots and Michael performed for Khali, her laughter spurring him on to bigger and wilder moves.

"Watch this, watch this," he squealed, spinning himself on the floor.

The witching hour disappeared. Steve returned home to pulsing speakers, laughing kids and a content wife, dinner ready. The music and movement lifted my mood and calmed my nerves. The kids equally delighted in the tunes, each other's enthusiasm and Mom getting-down.

During first chakra, I had created silence as often as

possible, craving its contrast to the noise of a house with young children. Silence wasn't going to cut it in *svadhistana*. There was a time for silence and a time for singing, and five o'clock proved perfect for the latter.

The dance floor became a place for us to connect, elevate our moods and shake off extra energy. Each day I glimpsed myself dancing in the mirror, I saw less structure and more flow. Until one day, nearing the end of the forty days in sacral chakra, I left the dance floor for the kitchen, not once having checked myself in the mirror.

Music returned rhythm to my family and my life. I learned to let go. I learned it from a five-year-old and a two-year-old and a breath practice and women around a table. Wave breath rarely occurred and yoga poses seldom flowed yet my vibrations and those of my family raised exponentially as the rhythm of yoga continued to infuse life off my mat.

14

A TUBFUL OF SECOND CHAKRA

One final hurdle remained. The one I assumed would be the easiest of all second chakra practices: creativity. Crafts with my kids seemed an easy way to tap into play, inner child and art all at once. Having young children gave me an immediate edge in exploring the creative aspect of second chakra.

It was *my* child that needed to play, the child inside me, not the ones beside me. They already knew how to play. It turned out I was out of practice and had no desire to start from scratch. I spent the forty days avoiding the part of second chakra that was supposed to be the easiest. I had yet to do creative projects with the kids that involved any degree of letting go of control: grabbing paint with our hands and flinging it everywhere, covering ourselves, each other, the cat, the house. My window to let go through creative expression was closing. The stickmen and smiley-faced suns drawn in crayon at the kitchen table stuck their tongues out at me. I performed the bare creative minimum.

My resistance stemmed from fear. If I popped the cork on creativity, allowing the free flow of unbridled play, I would have a huge clean-up project. The kids would think they could do it anytime and anywhere, and it wouldn't conform to how a responsible parent should act. Honestly, it had been so long since I knew how to be a kid, to lose control in a not-involving-alcohol sort of way, that I think my biggest fear was I genuinely didn't know how. What if I had no creative talent and cracking that bottle open only proved it was empty?

I had spent hours in the fields as a kid, building speed bumps out of dirt for our mini bikes and tunnelling mazes of snow forts in giant drifts. I returned home one day with one soaking wet socked-foot and one rubber boot, the other abandoned after countless attempts to retrieve it from the mud. I wove hook rugs and wrote and sketched for hours. When had I become *so* mature that I outgrew the ability to get lost in play and art?

As a last ditch effort, in the eleventh hour, I took up the tub crayons during the kids' bath time, determined to break through my boundaries and deny the inner critic the opportunity of saying, "that's not good enough, you are *not* creative, you are *not* talented, *you* are not original." It was time to disintegrate the pattern of safe behaviour. I didn't want the perfect piece of art, I just wanted to not do the same thing I'd been doing for so long.

The kids took up the task quickly without a thought to design, scale or reality. I jumped in before all the tub real estate was taken. As they developed the sides and back of tub town, I claimed the wall above the faucet.

Yes, it was like a homework assignment, but I closed my eyes, exhaled any preconceived ideas and pressed the bright blue crayon to the fibreglass. It glided across the smooth surface. I forged a flower, then another, changing the landscape. Finally, I set down my crayon and perched on the edge of the toilet seat cover. I had jumped my own fences and broke free of the stickmen and smiley-faced suns.

Abstract vines flowed into shapes and swirls that circled the taps and spout. Tiny blue flowers blossomed from the vines and spirals spun around the faucet. There was letting go; there was flow. The clean-up required considerable elbow grease and, surprisingly, after my successful artistic exertion, I had a limitless supply.

The atmosphere in my home transformed as I transformed. Issues continued to surface, yet the dance, music, drawing and singing helped ease the mood and shift perspective, allowing me to let go of what didn't matter. Still, the blocked emotional expression, and my denial of it, remained.

The work, the inquiries and the exercises from the year in yoga so far acted like a tidal wave gaining force and ground on the emotional dam I had spent years constructing. With complete destruction certain, the only questions were: When? and Would there be casualties?

"When I let go of what I am, I become what I might be."
~Lao Tzu

PART III

SOLAR PLEXUS CHAKRA

IGNITE

It takes friction to start a fire,
and awareness to not burn yourself.

15

THE DARK BEFORE THE DAWN

hird chakra gathering loomed. Alora emailed the group. She included the email address for one of her yoga teachers, Gurmukh Kaur Khalsa, and instructed each of us to send off a request to Gurmukh for a personalized forty-day meditation practice for the duration of third chakra. Alora also requested confirmation of those wishing to attend a two-day retreat in the Rockies of British Columbia instead of our usual day retreat at Sacred Forest Lodge.

I looked up the directions online and browsed the retreat's website. The site's photos boasted of tall trees, majestic mountains, a medicine wheel and a large mountain river. The website listed workshops for wellness, healing, writing, inspiration and personal growth. The property oozed retreat: well off the beaten path, no shopping or services nearby, and accommodations in cabins or teepees by the river. If I chose the teepee, my "ensuite" would be a shared outhouse thirty feet away. For a stay-at-home mom planning a night away from the kids, a fabulous spa and luxurious linens should have been in order, not bug netting and a wooden crapper.

I emailed Anna to gauge her reaction to the invite. We decided if we were to do the retreat we might as well experience the adventure of it. We chose the teepee by the river.

"You know," Anna caught up with me via phone, "fire walking could be a real possibility. They have it listed on their website and fire *is* third chakra."

Her logic seemed sound and I tried not to let my imagination get the better of me, or rather my fear, which, as it turned out, was the main emotional aspect of third chakra.

I clicked on the tab marked *Fire Walking* and read the details. I watched a YouTube video linked to the site and then did something I probably shouldn't have: I googled fire walking and injuries. I didn't have to look very hard to find a fire walking incident that sent six people to hospital with burns.

If I was nervous before I read the article, I was completely terrified after. I made up my mind not to participate before I even knew if it was part of our itinerary. I joked with Anna: "*Promise not to give away my location when I hide in the bushes during fire walking ceremony.*" I stood firm; I would not walk on hot coals. Period.

The next detail of the retreat, after location and lodging, was the date. For the first time, I struggled with my commitment to attend every gathering of the year in yoga. That particular weekend was full: Khali's second birthday, Michael's invitation to a friend's party, and my sister and brother-in-law hauling in their unwanteds for a garage sale at our house. I felt I was bailing on family commitments left, right and centre in order to honour a commitment to myself. I mostly struggled with Khali's birthday. I felt selfish taking the weekend to do something for me instead of celebrate her.

I was stuck between second and third chakra emotions: guilt and commitment. I decided to cast them aside and looked at the situation bereft of the emotions. At two, Khali wouldn't care which day we celebrated her birthday, it was me who made a big deal about the party. Steve was quite capable of transporting Michael to and from a friend's birthday party, and if my sister wanted to sell her things at my home, it didn't require my supervision. I let go of the need to control and contribute to every aspect of life around me. We pushed the party to the following weekend and I committed to third chakra retreat.

I figured a jump on the packing was a good idea, in case life got busy, so I gradually packed up the many items required for the stay. Alora always started with a simple list of requirements and four or five emails later I had packed up half the house and scoured the city for crystals or oils.

Anna and I decided to travel together, excited about the three-hour drive to catch up. We planned to drive past Banff, where we met nearly fifteen years earlier, and then head on to grab tea and pastries at our favourite bakery in Lake Louise. After that, it would be on to the retreat, but not before I searched the nearest town for the cleanest wash-room to make one last comfortable stop before the teepee and the outhouse.

Each aspect of third chakra made its presence known in my pre-retreat preparations. I argued with Steve the night before, leaving me exhausted and depleted. I experienced gripping, irrational feelings of fear, even panic, over leaving my children for the weekend. What if something happened to me? I felt like I was saying goodbye for the last time even though I knew it made no sense.

I tried being present in the moment and not letting my thoughts jump ahead to "what ifs". I tried logic but I had this nagging illogical certainty that I'd never see them again, that I wasn't coming back from the retreat. Fear, hostility, anger, doubt, all third chakra feelings: fiery emotions.

Since the kids were born, it fascinated and disturbed me how I could imagine all sorts of irrational scenarios where something terrible happened to one of them. When Michael was an infant, nightmares and daymares of the cat attacking him consumed me, which was baffling since anyone who's seen my cat can attest: he's a generous eighteen pounds of docile feline.

I suddenly feared for my own well-being, as the thought of leaving them without a mother equally scared me. And I feared for my husband's well-being for the same reason. Parenthood was a game-changer and there was no coach to brief me on the plays before I went on to the field. I remember a pep talk in the dressing room where we learned to feed them, change them, dress them and administer necessary medication, but where was the strategizing on keeping myself cool, calm, centred, rested, confident and assured? The emotions surfaced the night before the retreat and although I was aware of them I felt powerless to do anything other than react.

16

THE LATE BIRD GETS INDOOR PLUMBING

I placed my considerable gear into the trunk of my car, stuffing it to one side to make room for Anna's and Sandra's bags. Sandra had emailed a couple days earlier, asking if she could carpool with us. I had wanted to spend the time with Anna, just the two of us, but Sandra's British wit was always welcome.

I drove the familiar route to the hamlet to pick them up. I'd offered to drive, as it satisfied my need to be in control of both journey and destination. The faces of Anna and Sandra mirrored my own: anticipation and escape.

Three women in a car for three hours produced no lack of conversation. We agreed early in the drive to use the time without kids to discuss subjects other than our kids. We all dearly loved our children, but we recognized the trap of being consumed by mommy-hood and expressing no outer (or inner) interests. When our dialogue occasionally drifted to a child, a well-placed throat clearing gently nudged a conversation course correction.

I exited the Trans-Canada Highway and pulled into the parking lot near the bakery at Lake Louise. We each made our selection from the assortment of delectable treats and transported them with our tea to a picnic table set among the trees, not far from river.

I had missed the smell of pine and spruce mingled with earth. I missed the mountains like I missed an old friend. The smell of the forest and the mountain air welcomed me in a familiar embrace. In one breath, I felt restored, grounded. I felt like I was home.

"Let's take a moment to sit in silence on the rocks by the river while we honour our *svadhistana* practice." Anna said.

We accepted her suggestion. I took up position on a large rock at the river's edge near a wooden footbridge. Both speed and temperature of the water posed a force enough to humble anyone. I dipped my hand into the river. The crystal clear and ice cold water constricted the blood vessels in my hand and I felt the sting yet held it there, staying with the sensation, feeling the river's numbing effect. It was a game of chicken I could never win.

I surrendered and pulled my hand from the water. I took a deep breath of mountain air. The emerald green of the trees gave way to blue, cloudless sky. I understood why they were called the *Majestic* Rockies; once again they held me. I sat, lulled by the river: its loud lapping drowned out all other noise - all but the whistle of the passing train headed into the city. The smell of campfire in the distance pulled me from my commune with the river and alluded to what lay just ahead of us. We returned to the car and continued on our journey.

I turned off the highway past the town of Golden, and our last chance at a flush toilet. A paved road led us away from the main flow of traffic and up the mountainside. Asphalt turned to gravel as we approached a T-intersection and stopped. A wooden sign hung on a telephone pole in the ditch, pointing us in the direction of the retreat. I turned to continue our meandering route. Trees lined the road, broken up by driveways leading to homes; sheds, corrals, abandoned old vehicles, miscellaneous tires, car parts and trailers, were all contained within the mountains that surrounded us.

We turned into a driveway marked with the retreat sign, twenty minutes ahead of the scheduled start time; yet we were the last group to arrive. Most had arrived the day before, an option that those of us with children couldn't entertain.

The garden looked to be under construction: mounds of dirt spilled out on to the grass and no fencing. The main lodge stood unfinished with unstained wood and partial porch. The upper level and back side appeared newer, perhaps additions to an existing building. The large sign etched with the property name, *Spirit River Retreat*, rested in the grass in front of the lodge, also unfinished.

"Great," I mumbled.

I pulled into an open space in front of the main lodge, expecting someone to meet us and show us where to put our things and meet the group. No one appeared.

We got out of the car and searched until we found a man in what appeared to be a wood shop in the main building. He turned out to be the owner of the lodge, Brent. He wasn't sure where we would be sleeping but told us to put our things in one of the cabins and join the rest of the group down by the river.

I drove farther down the driveway and parked the car opposite a two-story cabin, more of a chalet. I popped the trunk and we pulled out our bags. We opened the door to the cabin and poked our heads inside just far enough to set our bags on the linoleum floor.

I peered around inside as far as I could see. A tiny kitchen with wood cupboards and full size appliances stood just off the entrance. A generous, open room housed the living and dining areas, showcasing the stunning mountain views from the large windows. The cabin was clean and tidy, not nearly as raw as I'd expected. A hardly comforting realization, since we had requested the teepee.

We headed by foot, further down the gravel road, assuming it led to the river and the others. We passed another two-story cabin, larger than the first, then down a hill where I could see the river in the distance and the top of the teepee: baby blue against evergreens. Difficult to miss, the big, beautifully crafted tent perched above the river bank. Equally difficult to miss: the dreaded wooden outhouse.

A couple people I didn't recognize stood near the entrance of the teepee. Anna leaned toward me and whispered. "Those must be the Sunday people."

I'd completely forgotten that Alora was combining the two groups for the retreat. Finally beginning to feel relative ease within my group, the reality of exploration among a new set of strangers reengaged my defences. My ego began to set up camp as sturdy and ceremonial as the large teepee.

I smiled at the people standing outside the tent, then pushed back the heavy flap to the entrance and ducked inside. My eyes adjusted to the low light as I looked around the interior at many familiar faces and some new ones. Four single cots, complete with mosquito netting, lined the perimeter and encircled a central fire. As it turned out, there was no room at the inn: all the teepee beds had been claimed the night before.

"Well, there you three are," Alora's voice sang out. "It's time to begin."

I thought we had arrived with enough time to settle. Evidently I was wrong. We followed Alora out of the tent; she quickly introduced the Saturdays to the Sundays, no time for chit chat. She led us down a path on the other side of the teepee, and I surveyed the monumental motel as I passed. Although the teepee was well-constructed and the cots raised off the floor looked comfortable enough, I felt relieved of my worry about relieving myself during our stay. I regained one creature comfort as I walked away from the rustic lodging.

17

LOST IN A LABYRINTH

Alora led us down the riverbank and onto the mud bed, flanking several small tributaries of the main river. She asked us to close our eyes while she said a few words: an opening ceremony and creating of sacred space. The retreat weekend formed a pivotal part of our year's journey in many ways. Mainly because it connected the work of all three lower chakras, allowing us, once complete, to move on to the upper chakras.

Alor offered gratitude to the river, the mountains and the energies that supported our journey. I didn't hear the rest of her spiel; I was busy brushing weird, thin-legged spiders off my legs. They seemed to appear from nowhere yet, as I stared at the muddy earth, it moved with the activity of creepy-crawlies. Others in the group stood, oblivious, holding their sandals, bare feet in the water or sinking into the mud. I kept my shoes on and, like an arachnid-fighting ninja, continued to return what seemed an endless barrage of spiders quickly back to the mud.

We followed Alora farther along the river to a clearing, the scar of a previous mudslide. She split the group in half for the first inquiry. Half of us would walk the labyrinth[1], connecting to Earth and root chakra, while the others spent time in an inquiry in water and second chakra. Then we would switch.

I fidgeted as I listened to her, feeling a bit dizzy and wanting to sit down someplace cool. It was hot. I was cranky from being rushed into the afternoon's events, without time for settling in or even a drink of water. *Go with the flow.*

Alora informed us that the entire outdoor earth and water inquiries were to be conducted in complete silence. Thank goodness the long car ride gave us the opportunity to visit. I shifted my weight from one leg to the other, impatiently listening to the instructions for walking the labyrinth.

"Enter consciously and walk toward the centre, looking inside yourself," she said. "Go deep within and take your time. Spend as much time at the centre as you need, then wind back out, feeling your expansion."

Sounded easy enough. *Not.* I hadn't a clue what she was talking about. Standing under the sun, annoyed by the heat, the tiny creepy-crawlies, and the lack of transition time, I wasn't sure how to go about looking inside myself and even less certain of the process involved in expansion. Was I to use my imagination or did it require large arm movements and twirling?

Alora led the other half of the group away and Anna left with them. I stood at the entrance to the labyrinth and steadied my focus. The sun beat down on me as I grasped for awareness in that moment, partly afraid of missing some profound opportunity with the experience and partly agitated from the heat. I was pretty sure my busy brain was not what Alora meant by *consciously entering*.

I stepped across the dried-mud start line. I exhaled as I

placed my foot down onto the path, as if I had just walked through a force field and into another dimension. I deliberately placed one foot in front of the other as I started down the narrow path, lined on both sides with rocks. Jill, a willowy blond, had entered ahead of me and stood a few feet in front. She moved slowly, far slower than me, so I adjusted my pace to keep distance between us. I recalled Alora's directions. *As I spiral in, I am to go inward.*

The path guided my steps around a tight curve and I no longer spiralled toward the centre, but instead away from it. I stopped and looked back toward the entrance. *Did I go the wrong way? Did I take the wrong path?* I checked the stones' pattern on the path, certain I had made a wrong turn. There was only one path and I was on it. Perplexed and annoyed with both the slow pace and the movement away from centre — which only indicated a longer trip to arrive — I carried on.

My thoughts prohibited me from silent union with the experience. *This is going to be a bust if I can't quiet my mind.* Then I recalled the questions I had asked myself. *Did I go the wrong way? Did I take the wrong path?*

No, there is only one path for me at this time and I am on it. The answer felt different than the questions. The questions had come from my thoughts, the all-too familiar voice in my head. They originated from my struggle. The answer, however, blew in like a gust of wind, seemingly from nowhere. Almost as if someone else had said it.

I laughed. I realized I didn't have to focus all my intent in the labyrinth. It was teaching me my lessons. I simply needed to pay attention.

The questions mirrored my life, showing me the behaviours and thought patterns that governed my decisions. *Did I take the wrong path?* was a common and crippling theme.

Trusting I was exactly where I was meant to be was a difficult process. And patience — to walk the path, knowing the destination would reveal itself in due time — was a quality I lacked.

One foot in front of the other. Enjoy the walk.

I continued farther along the path, which sometimes led toward the centre and sometimes veered out to the edge, only to turn again toward the middle. I grew comfortable with the pattern as it became familiar, like I was on to its little game. Once more, I noticed Jill ahead of me at a different point in the labyrinth. *How did she get all the way over there, so far ahead of me? We weren't that far apart at the beginning. It makes no sense.*

Questions flowed and answers followed. It was as if I were in conversation with the labyrinth itself. *Why am I concerned about where someone else is?* Focusing on my own path, and my place on that path, was also something with which I struggled in life. The labyrinth mirrored my issues. Life wasn't a competition. It wasn't a race. *She is where she is, and I am where I am.*

Eventually I got to where she had been, physically. Although we stood in the same place, I knew we experienced unique lessons. The labyrinth taught each traveler what they needed to know.

I finally reached centre, almost. I lifted my gaze from the path to see a labyrinth traffic jam. A small group congregated near centre awaiting their alone time in the middle. It was difficult not to race toward it, but instead, to slow down and appreciate the remaining few steps along the path. Realizing I needed to wait for everyone to have their turn was a letdown. All that work to get to centre and I couldn't float gracefully into it.

Starting a family, though one of the greatest joys of my

life, had also forced me to pause. Rather than resent the fact that my career was on hold, or my personal pursuits weren't front and centre, or try to cram everything in at once, it was time for me to accept the pause. It was time to simply look around and take a breath; to enjoy standing right where I was on my path.

The labyrinth asserted that life was not a race. The first one to the centre didn't win anything. Rather, she may be disappointed to find she had squandered the journey. Absorbed in contemplation, I awaited my turn.

In my early twenties I had waited tables and managed restaurants and bars, and knew that if wait staff focused on the tips, they would always be unsatisfied with their earnings and their work. I knew that if I focused on service, enjoying my conversations with diners and coworkers, the tips flowed freely, as did my satisfaction with both earnings and work. Basically, if I worked solely for the money, the money didn't come and neither did my happiness.

Able to apply my own bit of Confucianism in the workplace, I failed to translate it into life at home with kids. My days consisted of a never-ending series of self-created *goals*, rushing from one target to the next with scant appreciation of the in-between. Make breakfast. Get Khali down for a nap. Plan the evening's class. Find an activity for everyone. Make lunch. Clean up. Get kids outside for fresh air. Shop for dinner. Find a program for them to watch so I can watch mine while I make dinner. Teach class. Get kids into bath and bed. Hope to get a few hours sleep before someone wakes up in the night. My days had felt like a numbing chain of goals to be accomplished, rather than a series of mindful steps taken along the path of my day. I often expanded the goal-setting further to rush through the baby years to get to the toddler years when, hopefully, sleep would come easier. Goal setting continued as my mind jumped ahead to get the kids into school to create more time for a career. In the meantime, I rushed through the week to get to the weekend.

I pushed through seasons to get to holidays, and holidays to reach a new year. The *now* that Eckhart Tolle referred to in the first chapter of his book — *the present moment* I'd read about on my bike — became clearer. I understood what it meant to live in the future, I continually lived in the future. I knew little of the present.

I looked up to see people leaving the centre. Upon their exit from the altar, I became aware that the path *in* was also the path *out* of the labyrinth, a detail undisclosed by Alora in her earlier explanation. With the path only wide enough for one traveller, we were forced to work together. The hugging began.

As those leaving squeezed past those entering the altar area, they hugged. I observed some long, intense holding. I braced myself for the series of embraces to come. Three men participated in the retreat and one walked the labyrinth with my group. I had just met John an hour before, and since we started our practices in silence, not much getting-to-know-you had occurred. I was not comfortable sharing an embrace with the male stranger.

I watched as he lovingly hugged Jill right in front of me; they shared a warm moment together on the path. Emotions appeared high as they both teared up. *How do I handle this tactfully?* I had no intention of joining the emotional display. As he approached, I side-stepped, reached out to him and used him as a prop to get by him. No actual hugging occurred. Awkward, but all I could manage at the time.

I was no stranger to hugging. I came from a family of huggers. Whenever we saw each, all my relations embraced in familiar hugs and planted cheek kisses. Outside of my family, hugging was not something I shared with just anyone. I considered it a personal act that I only shared with those I trusted.

My meditative bubble burst, I waited impatiently until Jill rose from her knees to leave the altar. We shared a mixed embrace — her completion of reaching centre and my drive to do the same. *Finally, my turn.*

Alora had instructed us, in one of her many pre-retreat emails, to bring an offering to leave on the altar, something significant to our journey. I *had* brought one of my note-books, with the intention of leaving a page from it. Unfortunately, with the lack of communication upon arrival, and the immediate start to the activities, I did not know to bring my offering with me to the river. My notebook sat, packed in my bags with my supply of chocolate, back at the cabin.

"Great." I sank. "I made it to the centre with no offering. Perfect."

I knelt down in front of the small earthy altar. Colourful crystals and gems, feathers, pendants and flowers adorned it. Tiny angel sculptures and carvings of hearts became its bones. As I scanned the items, an unfamiliar emotion crested: an acknowledgement of the sacredness of the place — a feeling of relief and being cared for — by who or what, I wasn't sure. I simply felt humble and peaceful, reverent and safe.

What can I leave? I wished I had brought my book as I sincerely wanted to offer something special, a gift to honour the place and the experience. I plucked a hair from my head, just behind my left ear, and tucked it under a rock in the altar. Tears welled up in my eyes as I was overcome with emotion. I could no longer see the altar. I blinked the tears away and wiped those that escaped down my cheeks.

Something other than sadness elicited the tears, an emotion whose origin escaped me. I would later come to know the beautiful and intense emotion as gratitude — foreign to me for so long, I had forgotten its sweetness. Maybe I never knew gratitude, not the depth I began to feel after that day and after each and every sacred experience to which I allowed myself to surrender.

I muffled a sniffle, and turned to begin the outward expansion. After that, I hugged every person I encountered on the path. All girls, of course. It wasn't hard, although it preoccupied a large portion of the second half of the experience for me. The process of expanding outward unfolded around me and I embraced it, as I did the women on my path.

I found out exactly with whom I was comfortable expanding outward. The girls all responded warm, open and friendly, until I came to one of them, that is, Lisa. Since she had joined our Saturday group in second chakra, I didn't know her well. I leaned in for a hug and she stood there, looking at me. Maybe I got it wrong. Maybe her sunglasses hid her eyes and she was looking elsewhere and not at me. Maybe she deeply engaged me in a moment of conscious pause and I wasn't aware of it again due to the shading of her eyes.

I *felt* the awkwardness, the uncomfortable gap like someone left hanging on a high five. After a few seconds, she leaned forward for half a hug. *Am I not good enough to receive your hug?* In that moment, I felt like an outcast. Perhaps I misjudged, or rather shouldn't have judged the situation at all. Or maybe I had just received a realization of how John felt when I had side-stepped him. Karma's a bitch. Whatever the reason, I got schooled on my interactions with others. Judgment, comfort, trust, fear, power, vulnerability, unity, community, tribe, security; lower chakra issues abounded.

Once I safely cleared the onslaught of hugs and silent exchanges, I found myself alone once again with the path of the labyrinth, this time the exit in sight. I felt unburdened, as if I had left a heavy load of emotions and thoughts behind in the centre of the labyrinth.

Almost giddy, something I hadn't felt in years, I practically floated along the path. I felt like twirling in circles. Why didn't I twirl? *Do it.* Too controlled and reserved in the group dynamic — not wanting to draw attention to myself — I managed a slow stealthy spin at one of the path's corners. Baby steps, I guess. And I exited the labyrinth.

I stood outside the perimeter, watching others make their way out. I contemplated how I'd felt most comfortable at the outer edge of the labyrinth, closest to the trees and mountains, and then the most touched at the altar, the deepest core. The most uncomfortable times occurred in between, unable to feel the safe company of the trees or cradled at the bosom of the labyrinth, but taking patient steps, feeling lost amidst others on the path.

My gaze shifted to the altar, bereft of kneeling worshipers. I reflected on the single strand of hair tucked under one of its rocks. With the hair, I left behind a small part of me — personal but also part of my shell, my impermanent self — captured at the core of the labyrinth like a malevolent spirit.

18

MY RUN-IN WITH THE HUMMINGBIRD

I headed for the water. Alora's instructions had specified to go to the teepee, then back to the cabin to change and grab mats for yoga. At least that is what I heard. She had then said to make sure to experience both the labyrinth (earth) and the river (water). I assumed we were to go to the river ourselves and spend time with water.

I had removed my sandals at some point during my walk in the labyrinth, deciding the packed mud offered a clean enough surface and bugs appeared scarce. The earth had felt cool under my feet and had comforted me in the hot sun. I stood outside the labyrinth, assessing the rocky terrain leading into the trees, toward the teepee. I decided to leave my shoes off and brave a barefoot experience with the earth on the way to the water. Cool, packed, silky mud; smooth, small rocks; soft mounds of grass; and the odd twig woke up my soles. The kid in me woke up, carefree in nature, unconcerned with hazards, real or imagined. I sauntered along with all the time in the world.

I came to a fork in the path between the labyrinth and the teepee. Alora must have forgotten to include "heading to the river before ending up at the teepee" in her instructions. I stood in the middle of the split path. One way led to the teepee and the other to the river. *Shit. Which way?*

A high-pitched chirp chirp followed by a long, high whistle interrupted my thought. It sounded like fireworks screaming into the sky just before they exploded. There it was again. I looked up to see a hummingbird. She darted overhead, made her powerful chirping sound and shot off, trailing the uncanny fireworks sound behind her.

She performed this dance several times above the path that led to the teepee. I caught a flash of red. It was difficult to focus on her since she moved swiftly. At one point she shot straight up in the air, so high she nearly disappeared from view. Sultry Yvonne approached from behind me and stopped dead in her tracks once she noticed the elaborate grandstanding. We looked at each other with wide eyes and big smiles, acknowledging the magic. Then off darted the hummingbird into the trees.

After such a display, I decided it best to follow her path, the one leading to the teepee. Thistles and small shrubs poked my tender tootsies. I slipped into my sandals.

I came to a second fork in the path — down to the river or up to the teepee — an opportunity to second guess my decision. *Am I on the right path?* My thoughts from the labyrinth replayed in my head. I recalled Alora's instructions. I knew she had said to go to the teepee after the labyrinth but I also knew she said to make sure to experience both earth and water. She must have been remiss in her instructions on the river. Coupled with the appearance of the second path, another opportunity to change directions, I altered my route and opted to dismiss the hummingbird's effort. I headed toward the river determined to

complete the second part of our assignment. Yvonne sauntered on to the teepee.

How many dancing, chirping, firework-shooting
hummingbirds does it take to get a message to a newly-
waking, over-analyzing woman? Evidently, more than one. I
reached the river bank and removed my sandals. I walked
through the riverbed clay and through the small channels of
flowing water, warmed by the afternoon sun. I marvelled at
the rocks: blue, orange, white, rainbows sparkling in the
water. The ice cold flow of the main river and the warmth of
her smaller streams played Nordic spa as I walked between
them.

I focused my attention and my senses on everything
around me, to have the *experience* with water, but it felt
awkward, as if the whole thing lacked direction and
purpose. I wandered around the banks and streams for a
while and, when I thought my time spent with the river
sufficient, I walked back to the cabin.

I collected my bags from their temporary storage and
headed to the cabin Alora had pointed out as our accommodations. She'd said to take our pick of one of several available beds. I pulled open the cabin door and climbed the
long, straight flight of wooden stairs to the upper level. I
checked out all the bedrooms and threw my bags into a
sweet little queen-bedded room with a door to a substantial,
covered, wooden deck overlooking the mountains and river.

For the rest of the afternoon I decided to enjoy the
larger, sunlit room before retiring to the twin-bedded room
next door where I would likely be chatting with Anna into
the wee hours of the morning. I placed my bags on the bed,
grabbed my box of chocolate wafers, paper and pen, and
headed out onto the deck where I sat among squirrels and
birds, enjoying nature, quiet, solitude, and cookies.

Shaded from the sun in a relaxing chair with a perfect snack and a bit of writing, uninterrupted and freshly inspired, I finally felt a sense of retreat. The mountain air invigorated me, the silence enveloped me, and I sank into both. I wrote about my encounter with the labyrinth, all that surfaced, and was just about to start on a new tangent when I heard Alora yelling in the distance.

She called for someone to return to the river, two names. I recognized my own. I was certain we were to meet in the main house next for yoga. Had I missed something? "For crying out loud," I muttered. "I just sat down."

"Stephanie!"

I shut the cover of my journal, tossed it and my open sleeve of cookies into my bag, and headed back down to the river, pissed off about being summoned to return to the heat and the group.

I quickly discovered that my initial assumption about instructions was wrong and, had I remained on the path of the red, dancing hummingbird, I would have ended up at the teepee like I was supposed to. I hadn't trusted my feelings or my fast-flying guide and had chosen poorly.

The behaviour of the hummingbird was not one I easily identified with: flighty and appearing to make random movements. I didn't respond well to, what seemed to me to be, a lack of control or reasoning. I wasn't used to making quick movements based on the rhythms of nature.

When I became a parent I began making decisions based on lengthy, internal debates that often included pro and con list making, research, previous track records and the possibility of success versus failure. When the pendulum came along, it provided my first reprieve from that exhaustive process. Then came hummingbird: beautiful, light, graceful and quick, with a dance and a song as well, asking me to follow her.

How could it be so effortless to move through life with skill and grace? Whether I understood or agreed with the foreign patterns and behaviour of the hummingbird, the truth was that this delicate creature had information that could have helped me if I'd chosen to trust and follow her.

"You missed the water." Alora stood between the paths leading to the teepee and the river.

"No, I spent my time with the river."

"No, love, you missed the water experience."

She insisted but revealed no further detail. Our conversation unfolded like an Abbott and Costello exchange where neither was getting anywhere but further frustrated as we defended our stance. Yes, I did. No you didn't. Yes, I *did*. No you *didn't*.

Then she grabbed my hand and started skipping, asking me to skip along with her. When we'd arrived earlier that day, I'd told her my back had flared up and the weekend's exercises might prove challenging.

"Do you remember skipping as a child?" She happily dragged me along by the hand, oblivious to my angst and pain.

"No skipping, no skipping," I urged. Finally, my frustration cut loose and because it was kind, compassionate Alora, it came out of me in tears instead of a current of anger. "My back is done. *I'm* done. I can't skip." Feet planted, I stood my ground, trembling, frustrated, and wiping tears from my face, which made me even more angry.

"I thought your back had healed."

Her inability to understand — no matter how many times I explained it — that my type of injury didn't just heal like a cut finger or broken bone annoyed me to no end.

Truthfully, I was tired of the injury and frustrated with my inability to heal it once and for all. But my injury served only as an excuse at the river. I felt like a scared child in a crazy three-ring circus: odd characters, strange performances, surreal sets. Lost in the crowd of awestruck circus goers, I needed a familiar face to reassure me.

At that moment, Anna emerged from the path in the trees, floating in a dreamy bliss after a meditative exit from the labyrinth. Our eyes met. My anger and frustration must have been written all over my face because Anna's expression turned from peace to serious business. She made a beeline for me and explained that there was an organized part of the water inquiry that I hadn't yet done. I was relieved that at least my good friend spoke my language and in that one simple sentence communicated what I needed to hear. She provided a connection to the familiar, ending the confusing debate with Alora.

Anna headed back up the path toward the cabin. I turned back to Alora, who led me to a rubber raft. "Step in and lay down," she said.

Gladly. Because, from what I could tell, I was going to be alone in the raft and that was exactly where I wanted to be, alone. I removed my sandals.

"Do I take my sandals in the raft or leave them here on the shore?"

"Leave them here," she replied.

I left the words, struggle, tears and anger behind with my sandals on the river's rocky edge. I lay down on my back in the raft, closed my eyes and sank into the rubber cradle.

There, I could forget my struggle with Alora. Allowing her to lead me through a year of deeply personal, often confusing and mostly uncomfortable experiences was challenging. I didn't understand why I couldn't relate to her.

19

ADRIFT ON THE WATERS OF EMOTION

Had twenty minutes passed? Thirty, forty? Hours? I had no idea. I melted into the raft and the river's fluid embrace. The waves lapped at the raft and lulled me to sleep. Like slipping in and out of a dream, my groggy awareness shifted to someone running along the shore, a quiet companion watching over me. The water delivered much needed and accepted therapy. I had little energy or desire to investigate further.

By the cadence of the steps on the shore, I surmised their task was a strenuous one; they seemed to run and then dig in and struggle for a bit, and run again. I welcomed their care. Like a baby releasing a fit of frustration and then lovingly rocked in the fluid arms of Mother Nature, I fell, exhausted, into sleep, my eyelids too heavy to open if I tried. I surrendered.

I felt someone leaning over me. I pried my eyes open; the crystallized remnants of tears encrusted my lashes. The daylight forced them shut again. I squinted into the sky, my vision blurry. As I focused on the form above me, a tanned and shirtless young man materialized.

Short, dark, tousled hair framed a handsome face with warm, dark eyes. His lean physique boasted his well-defined muscles; sweat glistened on his skin in the strong rays of the afternoon sun.

Where am I? Am I dreaming? Watching a movie? I was fuzzy. Perhaps the heroine has washed onto a foreign shore after drifting for days, and is rescued by an exotic stranger. I felt better, calmer and peaceful, as if I'd been asleep for days. I wanted to remain in that state, awash on the new shore, in the company of a quiet stranger who knew nothing of me. A fresh start and a new place.

I sat up in the raft and looked around at the tree-lined river bank. I realized I had *no* idea where I was. The appearance of Brent from behind the raft provided comfort and yet disappointment in knowing that I was still on the property and part of the retreat. The two men helped me out of the raft. Disoriented, I couldn't see anything familiar in the surroundings except, of course, the fast-flowing river.

"Which way to the lodge?" I croaked out the words through dry throat.

Brent pointed the way. My bliss proved brief as I realized I must make the long walk back to the lodge with no shoes. *What the hell?!* Alora said it was okay to leave them behind. Had she not done the exercise herself? The terrain between me and the lodge was as hostile as my emerging feelings for Alora. I became a product of that environment with every step.

"We can carry you back in the raft, Cleopatra-style," Brent kindly offered.

I declined, feeling that would be a huge burden for two guys in the heat and terrain, and quite an imposition since I hardly knew them. I could make my own way back. I stubbornly but politely rejected.

"No problem," I lied, "nice day for a walk."

For fuck's sake. I carefully chose each step on the twisted, prickly, riverbank ground cover. I tried to think there was a purpose to the barefoot journey. *No sense being upset, enjoy the scenery and stop stewing.* But each step between the lodge and where the raft landed reminded me of the discomfort of the journey.

I alternated walking in the river against the icy current until my numb extremities could no longer bear the cold, with walking on the land as long as my feet could stand the stabbing of the thistles. Fuelled by anger and fierce independence, I returned to the retreat, my sandals and my cabin.

I stomped up the stairs and into my queen-bedded room with the mountain view. Finally, a chance to gather myself for a few moments, remove the thistles from my feet, and steady my nerves and my temper. The cabin door swung open and someone yelled up the stairs, "Hey, Stephanie, yoga's starting!"

FUCK!

20

HOT YOGA

Yoga mat in hand, I felt an overwhelming desire to beat it against a nearby tree. *Retreat, my ass.* Extreme heat and exercise never agreed with me. I headed to the yoga room at the main lodge to begin our practice.

The others appeared ready for a leisurely yoga class. I was ready for a boxing match. It took all my focus to work through the first fifteen minutes of the session. The heat in my face grew as I stewed about the painful hike, the constant rushing from one place to another, and the fact that everyone else seemed oblivious to this hectic "retreat" schedule. Was I the only one living a fiery experience? Was everyone else in a blissful bubble? It was hard not to get up and walk out of the room. *No drama. Hold it together. Do not let the memory of fire retreat be about drama.*

Alora set the tone for fire yoga. "For our third chakra asana practice, we will perform nine sets of twelve heart presses." Basically, one hundred and eight yoga push-ups, separated by brief postures to flush the lactic acid.

The entire group groaned in dismay. I felt relieved. I

welcomed the opportunity to channel my hostility and frustration into a form I knew and embraced: the push-up. Finally, familiar territory.

I efficiently pumped out all nine sets from my toes, the thought of dropping to my knees didn't even register. I exhausted every bit of negative energy I held, forcefully directing each breath from my body with every powerful exertion upward. Focus replaced anger as I turned my attention from recent events to counting off all one hundred and eight push-ups.

I released my body to the mat, lying on my stomach, forehead sticking to the cool padded surface. The heat dissipated from my body and my mind. A familiar fatigue sighed through my skin. Finally, I was ready to engage in the remainder of the yoga practice, which proved to be restorative.

I worked my body in the poses, paying attention to form and technique while adjusting the postures to protect my aching back. I even enjoyed the twenty-minute guided meditation at the end of the session, although I needed to perk up my ears to hear Alora's voice over the snoring. Lying on my mat, my back too sore to fall asleep, I focused on her words as I shifted from one hip to the other to alleviate pain.

"Third chakra ... fire chakra ... *manipura,* Sanskrit for *city of jewels.* This is the fire in your belly. Drive ... desire ... commitment ... all live here. Let the luminous yellow of *manipura* envelop you."

Several hours and myriad events had passed since I had arrived at the retreat, and I finally felt ready to proceed with the weekend. A lot of heat — fiery emotions — had been generated and burned off. It was as if layers upon layers of anger — stored over months, maybe years, maybe an entire lifetime — spewed forth, cooling into new earth.

21

FUEL FOR THE FIRE

I filled up on vegetarian lasagna, salads, spelt and potato buns, and chocolate almond torte with fresh raspberry coulis. The main lodge may have appeared rustic but the food was vegetarian gourmet. The day's heat, in its many forms, had burned a lot of calories, and the nourishment replenished my energy and steadied my nerves.

We returned to the teepee for Brent's explanation of the evening's activities. Brent stood at least six feet, if not taller, with a lean, tanned frame sculpted from the labour of tending the property. He had a comfort with the outdoors and the land, and a relaxed, simple demeanour. He was a combination of Jed Clampett and a California surfer.

"It's entirely voluntary. I never know if I'm gonna cross until it's time to go." Everyone listened as Brent shared his history with the fire-walk and where it all started for him. He mentioned the temperature of the coals would reach eleven hundred degrees Fahrenheit.

One of the women from the Sunday group sitting oppo-site me, kept repeating "eleven hundred degrees" like a

stuck record, to which I finally replied, "It's only a number."
Nice response from the one who had already decided not to
walk it.

That was the plan; yet, as I sat on one of four blanket-
covered cots, certain the majority of the group would not be
walking on the coals, something happened. Something
inside me churned, a wave of inner strength, of fearless-
ness, desire. The strongest sense of conviction suddenly
stood up inside me, fist raised in the air. I *would* walk
the fire.

*Why wouldn't I? I have come all this way, not just to the
retreat but here, to third chakra, having already struggled and
triumphed through the first two. More than eighty days into the
year in yoga and not a day had passed that wasn't filled with my
hard work, commitment and courage.*

The challenge lay at my feet and I could not pass it up.
*What is the worst that could happen? I could burn my feet. In
which case, I'll seek treatment and eventually they'll heal.* At that
moment, I was poised to risk injury for what seemed like a
momentous event. I chose to walk the fire. I sat up taller on
the cot. A grin burst from my lips. I accepted the challenge
like a brave knight, confident in my mission.

Brent explained a few planned exercises before the main
event was to begin. The first of which was building the fire;
an important and sacred task considering the logs' responsibility to my tender toes. "We're gonna build this in silence.
And reverence. And take as much time and respect as
it takes."

Brent led us out of the teepee and into two lines, facing
each other, between the riverbank and the teepee. He
handed each piece of wood from a substantial pile to the
person at the end of the lines, who, in turn, passed the wood
to the next person and down the lines to the location of the

bonfire. I practically kissed the first few pieces: *Please be kind to my feet.*

After several pieces of wood made their way to the bonfire location, Anna and I got goofy, reminiscent of the days of artist receptions at the gallery in Banff. Nervous anxiety gave way to laughter. Antics ensued. Standing side by side in our line, we used the pieces of kindling as musical instruments while we strummed log guitars. We cradled log lovers that we kissed and fondled, offering exaggerated tongue when no one was looking. Whatever the wooden shapes conjured, we obliged.

We passed the final pieces to Brent, who laid them on the massive bonfire frame. He lit the wood that held our signatures, and perhaps a little residual saliva. As the blaze took hold, we returned to the teepee where Brent handed us each a board one square foot across and half an inch thick.

"Draw or write on one side of the board whatever holds you back in life. And on the other side, make two lists. One list of what you wanna let go of and the other what you wanna bring in. Use words, pictures, colours, anything you like."

After eighty days of wading through my personal junk pile, I held a pretty clear idea of what I wanted to let go of. Although the process exhausted me at times and often the ups and downs of eurekas and ah-ha moments paired with failures and roadblocks made me question the point of it all, the ah-ha moments were too compelling to deter the process of further investigation.

The day's hostile takeover shed light on the struggles in my life and I listed them on the board: judgment, independence at all costs, criticism of myself and others, indecision and false power. Anger. I was ready for a gentler way: ease, effortlessness, community, creativity, laughter, joy and abundance. To the list I added the one thing I had resisted including in my inquiries until then: my back and the inability to heal myself. I surrendered it with the rest of my discards.

We sat in groups of three to discuss our wooden works of art, sharing their meaning and impact on our lives. Tears trickled and laughter flowed as we talked, held by the mountains, soothed by the river's voice and washed by soft rain. We concluded our comments and gathered around the fire. Sparse clouds rushed the mountain valley. The droplets of rain, no match for the bonfire, cleansed my tear-stained cheeks as the sun sank slowly between the peaks of the mountains, sparking the clouds on its descent. A somber atmosphere descended.

Brent stood at the foot of the bonfire, behind two tree stumps about waist high and several inches apart. He placed his piece of wood on top of the stumps. He raised his hand in the air and brought it down swiftly to slice through the wood. I perked up, excited by the opportunity to break my board. I had studied martial arts at seventeen and the guys I trained with delighted in creative ways to break boards: hands, feet, head, spinning kicks, jumping off another guy's back. I felt confident about the challenge.

I walked straight up to the stumps, board in hand, first to follow Brent. I placed my board on top and thought about all I was breaking through. I took a deep breath. The exhale trembled. Remembering the wise instructions of my past karate kin to not stop at the board but strike as though my target lay on the other side, I broke straight through the wood. Triumph. I retrieved the broken pieces from the ground and added them to the fire. Beaming with satisfaction, I returned to my place in the group.

Empowered, others broke through their boards one after

another. Several girls, however, had a tougher go of it. A few boards weren't broken and a couple boards even did the breaking. Two girls ended up days later with casts or braces on their wrists.

We stood around the fire, the energy of the air elevated from the board breaking. Brent handed out arrows: long wooden ones with smooth metal tips and feathered ends. I looked around for the bows but found none.

"Where are we going to break these, over our heads?" I asked, half joking, of Alora and Anna standing next to me.

A quick "You'll see," from Alora let me know it was going to be much more interesting than that.

Brent returned to the foot of the fire where he placed the metal-tipped arrow in the softest part of his throat, the area just above the V notch. He then placed the feathered end against his partner's outstretched hands so that the arrow suspended between them. He slowly leaned into Monica, who stood strong. The metal tip pushed against Brent's throat until the arrow's shaft bent and then snapped.

I turned to Anna, exuberant about the exciting new challenge. The look of terror on her face spoke volumes. I walked up to Brent, arrow in hand, and asked if he would steady the other end for me. Attempting the exercise for the first time, I wanted a professional assistant. He pressed against the arrow as I placed the tip into my throat, intensely aware of its intimidating presence.

I tried to relax as the metal point choked my breath. A surge of adrenaline drew panic to my chest. I leaned in fast to release the suffocating hold on my throat. The arrow bent at first, cutting off my airway, then straightened again. Confused at the misfire, I realized I must have backed off in fear when I felt the pressure escalate, the arrow's tip threatening to pierce the very source of my breath. I quickly leaned in with full commitment to the sharp snap of the shaft. My heart raced.

I tossed my broken arrow onto the fire, as I had done with the split boards, high on adrenaline and pride. Alora and Brent yelled out, "No!" and I quickly retrieved the pieces before they caught fire, not thinking how the metal tips would have acted as branding irons on the soles of our feet during the subsequent fire-walking.

I walked back to Anna, leaned over and said, "That was for you. It's easier than it looks. Commit."

She marched straight up to Brent. *Snap.* Each person in turn broke their arrow. Alora handed me her camera to capture our successes, bonfire blazing in the foreground, arrows snapping in the distance. Individually, we faced our fears. Collectively, we built momentum — a momentum imperative to carry us across the fire.

22

THE TUNNEL OF LOVE

Our next activity terrified me. Give me board breaking or arrow snapping any day. Anything but this. We formed two lines, shoulder to shoulder, one line facing the other.

"Each person will slowly walk through the lines, eyes closed, and receive love from the others. If you are in the line, you may wish to stroke the hair of the person walking through or hold their hand, offer loving words, compliments, affection, hugs ..."

I froze. I welcomed another arrow in the throat — or, quite honestly, to the head — a return to the icy river, anything other than what Alora described. I stood, crippled at the thought of walking down the line. I didn't know most of the people, three of whom were men. I was not interested in a forced affectionate moment and would rather walk on hot coals than be subject to the fondling of strangers.

I was finally developing a comfort level with sharing life's disappointments, fears, struggle and triumphs verbally with the group. A full-on public display of affection with these people was a leap I wasn't ready to take. Distraught, I took a place near the end of the line, prolonging the inevitable.

I offered reassuring pats on the back or arms of those travelling through the tunnel of love (there, there, you'll make it out okay, hang in there), more preoccupied with how quickly the line was moving than my offering of affection to the other. Most people lingered, lapping up the attention, seemingly unable to get enough, smiling and languishing in the tunnel.

My turn came, the end of the line. I closed my eyes and stepped forward, every part of my body clenched tight. My eyes began to leak. They weren't tears of sadness or joy, not the tears of frustration I cried when resisting Alora's skipping, and certainly not the tears of gratitude I experienced in the labyrinth. They were tears of extreme discomfort, tears of aching, of fear, of others penetrating the walls I had spent a lifetime building. They rolled unstoppable down my face. I needed space, room to breathe. My throat closed, my fists clenched, I reluctantly took one step after another, wanting to race through to the end, unscathed.

As I moved rigidly through the human channel, trying to slow both my pace and breath, I heard Yvonne's soft, melodic voice penetrate my closed ears, "You are a beautiful Hawaiian princess." I continued forward to hear Caroline, "A warrior princess." Somehow the words reached me, and the lineup of love became less horrible.

The words, spoken softly from the heart, affected me. They conjured images of strong women. I identified with the warrior — training hard, pushing myself to be better, stronger, more capable. The soft, radiant manner of a princess — creating beauty through grace and femininity — I hadn't seen in myself since before children.

The thought of the energies in balance: graceful power,

yielding strength, skillful ease, and tireless kindness, suggested a new way of relating. The rigid way I had been living needed to yield to a gentler method. Like the pain in my back conveyed, if I didn't learn to bend, I was soon going to break. I felt the sincerity behind the words spoken to me and in that brief moment was thankful to those two women who offered their kindness when all I wanted to do was create space between myself and the group. Still, after they spoke, I rushed through the remainder of the love line to temporarily slip into the shadows of night as the group continued hugging and loving by the fire.

23

OUT OF THE PAN AND INTO THE FIRE

B rent grabbed a rake, walked up to the bonfire and combed down the blaze, taming it into a hot bed of red coals. As we encircled the blazing bed, I waited for the chanting, dancing, meditation or whatever primal ritual would put us in the frame of mind we needed to spur our crossing of the coals.

"The first crossing is to get rid of the things you no longer want in your life," said Brent. "The return walk is to bring in the things you want." Brent stepped onto the coals and walked across and back. "Next."

I stared into the oscillating red and black of the crackling coals, stunned. *Seriously? No build up? No working up the courage or summoning forth some kind of brute ancestral energy to carry us across?* Then I realized that was exactly what we'd been doing all night. We broke boards with our hands, arrows with our throats, hugged our friends farewell in the tunnel of love and now into the fire we go. All the work suddenly felt insufficient to propel me across the sparking bed.

I turned to Anna, "I did you a solid with the arrows by going first. It's your turn to return the favour."

And with that, Anna walked up to the bed of coals, walked across, turned, and walked back. I watched to see if she was doing the burnt-foot dance but, no, she seemed fine. *Thanks, Anna*. It was one of the many reasons we were sister cats. We each had our strengths and what was troublesome for one of us came easily for the other.

Up I headed toward the coals. I walked directly and quickly, so as not to lose my nerve. I wanted to go right after Anna but John beat me to it. I was consumed in my own world, and not engaged in witnessing his crossing, as I waited at the top of the bed for his return. *Breathe*. I could hear someone inside me whisper. *Breathe*.

John stepped off the hot bed and I stood looking across the coals. I took less time to steady myself than I did with the board breaking. There was no hesitation, no thought. I took a breath. I know I took a breath. The last thing I remembered was that breath and feeling the heat on my feet, and suddenly I stood on the other side facing the coals once again. A blur, a portal through time. *When did I cross?*

The journey back loomed before me. I hadn't thought about the first crossing. Not even what I was supposed to think about letting go of in my life. I just took a breath and leapt. On the opposite side I paused — to think. *What was I supposed to remember on the way back across the coals? How did I cross so easily? Why am I still standing here?*

My body shook. My breath stuck. I couldn't move. I had to propel myself forward before I lost my nerve to return. I launched across the smouldering bed. My last step kicked up coals with my heel, sloppy step. I felt the sting on the sole of my foot.

I made it to the other side of the bed, a feat in itself. How

I arrived there spoke volumes. The way I had been living my life the past several years, filled with endless debate and struggle in my mind, often resulted in emotional and physical paralysis. I had been creating my own perceived misery for years, constantly questioning my path and actions, second-guessing my responses and choices, crippling my ability to take the next step. I had allowed fear to rule my life.

It was never about whether I would raise children, or if I would get sick; would I be successful, would I be happy, would dinner get made, would I get any sleep at night? It was about *how* I chose to have the experiences. Did I want to continue to travel through life with a head full of self doubt, criticism, judgment and fear? Or was I ready to leave it all in the ashes under my feet, take a breath and begin moving in a new way — one that allowed me to flow through life with less resistance and more ease, grace and joy? Like a warrior princess. It was time to cultivate the wisdom of all the battles I had fought — real and imagined.

I headed directly to Anna for a hug. We did it. We walked the fire. My foot stung. I knew that last step had burned me: a *kiss from the fire.* I remembered the phrase from the article I had researched on fire-walking — not comforting after the fact. I repeatedly shifted my weight into new cool grass to soothe the sting.

Everyone walked the fire that night. Many returned to the bed for seconds. I even think Gabriella crossed a third time. I remember her slow and deliberate ceremonial dance: one foot in front of the other, hands in the air, grinning like the Cheshire Cat. We did it, together. I had no interest in a second walk. I was more than satisfied with my experience.

Hugging, hooting and hollering began. A young girl, hula hoops in hand, joined us by the coal bed. A dull grey trail of ash remained. She lit a hoop on fire and started to twirl, the celebration underway. Many in the group attempted the fiery hula hoop while others shared in their triumphant tales of fire-walking. Drums began to beat. Music accompanied the drums.

I limped to the river on my heel, to wash away the soot before returning to the cabin to assess the damage. I saw the results of my sloppy step in the light of the cabin: three blisters. One minor, one larger, and a particularly painful one with burnt embers embedded in it like silvery-black slivers. I sat tall on the night stand, the lamp pointed at my foot, using Anna's tweezers to pluck the embers.

The pain was intense and the throbbing would be hard to sleep through, but I had walked across the coals and that accomplishment outweighed the pain. The blisters were my badge of courage, of facing my fears and rising above them. I walked the fire, something I thought I would never do. The blisters would heal and eventually disappear but the effects of the experience would last a lifetime. Third chakra, fire chakra, and my inner city of jewels, glowed as brilliantly as the embers had under my feet when I crossed to the other side and back again.

24

THE MASK OF A WARRIOR PRINCESS

S leep did not come easy that night. Even as I breathed through the searing pain in my foot and started to settle in bed, the sound of the crickets was deafening. Once the early morning birds joined in, sleep proved impossible. Finally, at five-forty, Anna and I started chatting. Yoga was scheduled for six-thirty, giving us plenty of time to linger under the covers.

Too tired to get up and too awake to fall asleep, we quietly talked, hearing no movement or noise from the others in the cabin. We revisited the details of the previous night's festivities in awe of the events we had shared and of our ability to rise to the occasion time and time again. We slowly crawled out of bed and dressed for the morning's yoga.

We stepped outside and into the calm of early morning in the mountains — the birds, the only sound. I inhaled the perfume of the Rockies, earth mingling with evergreens. The smell and cool morning air were Nature's coffee. We walked to the main lodge, yoga mats in hand, while others emerged from the cabins and between the trees. We silently converged upon the yoga room.

I opened the door. A wave of warmth and the smell of wood fire greeted me. Alora tended a black, metal fireplace in one corner of the room, cajoling the burning wood with a long iron poker. The large space was toasty and cozy, with wood walls and vaulted ceiling. Windows along two walls invited the morning light and green trees. I placed my mat on the carpeted floor and sat down.

Despite everyone's presence, the room remained quiet, each of us half awake. We flowed dreamily through the gentle postures. In spite of my sleeplessness, both my body and mind were energized and I enjoyed the morning practice followed by a twenty-minute guided meditation, once again difficult to hear over all the snoring. Evidently sleep hadn't come easy to *anyone*.

We took the opportunity at the end of our practice to string our commitment bracelets for third chakra. Alora pulled a variety of citrine beads from her bag, along with elastic.

"I must have forgotten to pack the string," she said as she searched her bag. "Those of you wishing to use string can wait and get some from me when we get home."

I didn't like the idea of an elastic bracelet when my others were tied onto my wrist with string but I knew if I didn't string it right then, chances were I wouldn't get around to it. I chose elastic. Why did what appeared to be my dominant chakra, end up being the one that I could remove at will?

We headed down to the river where Brent and Monica greeted us once again. I completely forgot about the sweat lodge until I was standing next to it. Monica, dressed in a long, ceremonial cotton gown, added logs to a fire in front of a small dome-shaped structure covered in an assortment of heavy blankets. The river flowed behind the dome, with a family of trees lining the bank between. Smaller than I expected, I wondered how the sweat lodge would accommodate all of us at once.

Monica instructed us on the attire we needed for the sweat: preferably a cotton night shirt or gown, but bathing suits or shorts and tank tops also sufficed. We returned to our cabins, replaced yoga attire with sweat lodge dress and ran back down the path to the river.

Laid out on the ground next to the lodge were squares of colourful cloth — maybe four to six inches wide — pieces of string and dried plant material. Monica asked us to gather around; she shared a story of prayer ties and instructed us on their design. I wasn't paying attention to the exercise. I don't recall where my thoughts were at the time but I know they weren't focused on the activity. Like a school kid not paying attention in class, I had to watch Sandra construct hers and quietly asked her to repeat the directions for me.

I sat on the ground, fumbling with the string on my tiny packet, trying to secure the offering inside.

"Why would someone wear makeup to a sweat?" Caroline's question interrupted my concentration and the silence of the group. I looked up to see her looking at me and realized I was the only one wearing makeup. I found the question confrontational, mostly due to the blunt manner in which she posed it. It came out of left field. *Why does she care if I'm wearing make up? Aren't we making prayer ties?*

When I woke that morning, dressed, applied makeup and pulled my hair into a ponytail, I wasn't thinking that we were hours away from a sweat lodge ceremony. I had never done a sweat. Was it her issue or mine? A bit of both I, suspected. She was the one who brought it up, yet I found myself reacting to it. Caroline, an older Scottish woman with long grey-white hair, stood, immovable, hands on hips, looking at me.

I paused as I considered my makeup motives. I felt more attractive with it, obviously. That was the reason for most appearance decisions: clothes, hair, makeup, jewelry. What I think bothered me about the question was, it pointed to the root of choosing to enhance my appearance. Was it purely to enjoy the way it made me feel or did it have more to do with my caring about how others saw me? Self-criticism surfaced as I analyzed the motivation behind a simple, habitual detail in my life.

Why does any woman wear makeup? Since our second chakra experience with our inner child, goddess and femininity, I became comfortable adorning myself with jewelry and flowing skirts, something I hadn't done since before the kids. Playing with my feminine side by wearing soft, flowing, frivolous garments and colourful jewelry made me feel softer, more playful, more creative. The garb emphasized a less prominent part of me.

But was I just playing dress-up? Did I need the garb to play the part? Of course not. A princess does not need to wear a gown to prove her virtues. Nor does a warrior need a weapon to show her courage. A warrior does, however, know that a mask is not worn to conceal or hide. A mask is worn to channel that part of her that part that already exists, and is needed in greater concentration for the task at hand.

My recent reunion with my feminine expression fell under attack, by one of my own tribe, no less. Defensive, the warrior nature rose in me as heat rose in my cheeks. Caroline's affront sparked a familiar fire. The truth was, no matter the motivation, to impress others or not, I remembered looking in the mirror that morning and feeling *really* good, shimmery lip gloss, defined eyes, swinging ponytail and all.

I needn't defend that to *anyone*. Well, except myself, who I began to see as the only one I needed to please. The tunnel of love from the previous evening resurfaced. It was Caroline who had called me a warrior princess. It was Caroline who challenged me in that moment, challenged me to get clear on who I was, challenged me to balance the warrior and the princess.

I chose a softer approach than my usual sharp retaliation. I allowed the heat to dissipate from my face as I took a deep breath and smiled. "It's a biodynamic brand of make-up," I said. "From Germany. I love it. I'm certain it'll outlast the sweat." I deflected her question and disengaged from the exchange.

As I finished my prayer tie, I briefly pondered Caroline's side of the question. We each held our own issues to address, our own mountains to climb. I understood how community helped us to bring the issues to the surface as each other's mirrors. The tricky part was acknowledging my climb and not reacting to someone else's mountain. I walked to the river, prayer tie in hand, bent over the fast flowing water and gently set my prayers afloat. I watched the small, colourful bundle bounce and bob, carried on the river's back.

25

MY MASK WEATHERS THE SWEAT

My heart beat faster. I shifted my weight from foot to foot, careful to avoid the tender underbelly of my blistered right sole. We gathered near the fire to hear Monica's instructions for the sweat. Nervous expression filled many faces. Others in the group mentioned how unbelievably hot it would get and I feared I might pass out or have to run for the outhouse. My bowels kicked in under extreme heat: one of the reasons I didn't like to exercise in it.

"If you find it too hot, you need to lay your head down against a cool patch of earth on the sweat lodge floor." Monica's confirmation of the heat only fuelled my anxiety.

She made it clear that should any one of us feel the experience too intense, we were to yell out "open the door" and Brent would help us to immediately exit the sweat lodge. The eagle feather snapped like a riding whip as it cut through the air around my body. Monica smudged me while I stood, awaiting my turn to enter the small, dark cave.

I ducked my head and crouched down to clear the doorway of the lodge. I followed others in front of me clockwise around the inside perimeter of the dome. We sat on blankets laid on the ground around a smooth deep pit: the navel of the sweat lodge.

I sat almost exactly in the centre of the group circling the dome, directly opposite the door, gazing across the navel. I looked around at how many people I would have to crawl over to make a run for the outhouse. Raised voices redirected my attention. Outside the door of the lodge, Brent and Monica discussed what appeared to be a serious issue with a member of the group. My anxiety seemed minimal compared to Sandra's apparent fear. Clearly the type of panicked discomfort that had gripped me in the tunnel of love, now consumed her outside the sweat lodge.

"You sit very near the door, and if things get too intense for you, I'll open it and you can leave." Brent worked to reassure her. Where I struggled with heat, Sandra's fear appeared to be more rooted in being in a dark, confined space.

Monica entered the lodge and sat next to me, slightly forward, at the edge of the pit. Sandra took up position on the edge of the doorway, her arms tightly hugging her knees in front of her as she sat on the ground, rocking quickly back and forth. Monica asked Brent to begin bringing in the lava rocks, which had been heating in the fire since the wee hours of morning.

Brent fished out four rocks from the fire with a pitchfork, feeding each one into the mouth of the lodge and the clay pit. Monica sprinkled herbs over each of the rocks. I didn't pay attention to what she added. My focus wandered to the proximity of the group members to one another, checking the walls and roof of the sweat lodge for creepy crawlies, and finding a comfortable position that didn't impose upon

Anna's space next to me or that of Monica's on my other side.

The heat of the rocks immediately warmed my face as Brent placed them in the centre from outside the dome. They sparked and crackled, danced and glowed red. Brent then pushed a large, silver bucket of river water through the door and crawled in after it.

Tight in the dome, we sat shoulder to shoulder or hip to hip, whichever way each of us could best adjust our bodies. Once we all settled, Brent poured the bucket of water over the glowing rocks. Steam spewed into the air. Brent set the empty bucket outside, resumed his spot at the entrance, and pulled the blanketed door flap closed. Darkness enveloped the group. The moist steam tickled my skin while I hoped no multi-legged intruders were mounting an attack on me in the dark.

Monica began to drum in the pitch black. Whimpering accompanied the beat. Soft cries near the door. Disoriented in the darkness, I followed the sound across the dome to Sandra. Whimpering became sobbing as the darkness spurred her distress. I felt certain her call for the door was imminent. Her sobbing increased. She held her ground as the drum beat slipped through the steamy air of the lodge.

My knee hit Anna's when I uncrossed my legs, searching for a more comfortable position. Monica's voice joined the drum to create sacred space for our experience. She called aloud to the spirits and the keepers of the tradition of the sweat, to those who sweated before us and those to come. The sobbing began to subside. Stillness filled the lodge and the first round of sweating and sharing began.

"If you use a spiritual name, please speak it before you share." Monica guided us through the intention of each round and then, one at a time, we shared something

personal in line with the intention. Apparently, no one in
our group used a spiritual name. One after another shared
in the dark, until...

"Creator."

I recognized Alora's voice.

"It is I, Hummingbird."

Well, that explains a lot.

The darkness freed me and I shared easily, relieved of
the gaze of others. Almost anonymously, I spoke my truth
into the blackness of the dome, listening, with no judgment,
to the voices that shared their truths in turn.

A dry heat was intolerable; I welcomed the hot steam. It
soaked into my skin, my pores, my lungs, hydrating every
cell. Trickling down my face, my neck, between my breasts,
it pooled in my hip creases. I wiped damp hair from my face
and absorbed the nourishing, deep treatment of Nature's
steam bath. The contrasting cool earth pressed against the
backs of my legs as I shifted position again. My shoulder slid
across Anna's as the water dripped off our skin.

My physical body detoxed while my mind cleared, with
no sight to stimulate chatter in my head. My spirit soared
with the depth of my sharing and those of the others. Purification. The victory over my anxiety belonged to the whole
group as did the victory of our sweat sister, Sandra, over her
deep fears of the darkness and the tight space. We soared
together.

At the end of each round, Brent opened the door. The
daylight blinded me and the summer air chilled my damp
skin. Many took the opportunity to leave the lodge and
jump into the icy, mountain river. I remained in my place in
the lodge. The dark, warm, moist cocoon comforted me and
I wanted the door closed so no heat could escape.

After the final round, upon the closing of the ritual, a

strong sensation gnawed at my body, more specifically, my belly. I was famished. As it was customary to fast before a sweat lodge ceremony, we hadn't eaten since dinner before the fire ceremony the night before — save for a handful of chocolate wafers I devoured sometime around midnight.

I emerged from the cocoon, lighter in both body and spirit, and took a deep breath of mountain air. The elements, the drum, the spirits, the ancestors, the sweat, the tradition, had created a transformational soup that left me feeling nourished.

We formed a line and hugged each other in turn — a truly joy-filled, sweaty celebration. I enjoyed *every* hug. As I embraced Brent, I assumed I would clutch and go, as I'd done with the other men. But Brent extended a hug as if he were gifting me a sacred space to be with whatever I needed in that moment, and however many moments I needed to be. There was no urgency to move on, only an honest, patient, connection with someone I had only recently met, no consideration to gender.

I floated off to my cabin to shower, dress and pack up my things — which I seemed to do at the speed of light. The promise and aroma of brunch hung in the air. And, like all experiences that weekend, the meal did not disappoint. A buffet of fresh, organic yogurt, muesli, fruit, pastries, jams and floral-infused spring water awaited us.

We lounged outside on the decks of the main lodge, devouring the delicacies, inhaling the fresh mountain air, bathing our faces in the sun, sharing laughter and enjoying the chatter of each other, and the mountain birds and squir-rels who awaited any leftovers. Everyone looked renewed. It showed on each of their fresh faces, in their smiles and the way they moved.

I left my seat in the sun and walked into the dining room to settle my bill with Monica. Lisa's voice surprised me.

"Your makeup looked great after the sweat. It didn't smudge at all. What brand do you use?"

At first I thought perhaps she was teasing me. Then I realized she was genuine. I'm not sure if her question was true curiosity or a show of support after Caroline's confrontation. It didn't matter. It felt honest and kind. Lisa and I had finally connected. I was learning how to be a part of a community and my community was learning how to be with me. Both my makeup and I had indeed survived the sweat beautifully.

I had entered the weekend with fears, uncertainty, self-criticism, rigid beliefs and ego. I left the weekend renewed, filled with a sense of belonging, self-acceptance, trust and new strength that came from a softer, gentler way of being in the world. The earth supported me, gave me a firm place to stand and a soft place to sit, supported my feet through the labyrinth, soothed my burns after the coals, and cooled my skin during the sweat.

The water sustained me, provided relief from the thistles on the long walk from the raft, cleansed my blisters after the fire-walk, provided the steam that purified every cell in the sweat lodge, and quenched my thirst on the hot summer days. The fire brought my fears to light and burned them away, clearing old patterns, beliefs and self-doubt; it heated the rocks that, combined with the water, enveloped me in the sweat lodge.

My foundation strong, the next forty days in fire chakra and, coincidentally, the heat of summer, would solidify my base, providing the platform to expand into the upper chakras. I knew there was more work ahead of me. Third chakra proved to be the seat of many of my issues. Pieces of me no longer existed, burned away in the fire, and I had tasted enough sweetness to know that the payoff was worth the work. There was no going back.

> "When you live in a community, you bump up against each other, and you really have to work on yourself."
> ~Venerable Thubten Chodron, from *Dakini Power* by Michaela Haas

PART IV

STUCK IN THIRD CHAKRA

TRANSFORM

Changing shape requires heat and pressure.
It also requires patience and perseverance.

26

YOU'VE BEEN GURMUKH'D

I returned home from the retreat to Gurmukh Kaur Khalsa's email: my personal forty-day meditation. The next email came from Alora, informing us third chakra term wouldn't last forty days. We were to break for summer and reconvene for fourth chakra in September, nearly *ninety* days later. *Crap.*

I flipped back to Gurmukh's email and opened the attachment. It was not what I'd expected. In fact, it didn't seem like a meditation at all. The practice began with an opening chant, then the meditation itself, which involved eleven minutes of controlled breathing and synchronized hand movements. The eleven minutes finished, another exercise of breath-holds and hand movements ensued, followed by one last chant to complete the practice. Meditation boot camp.

I felt confident in my daily practice. I could sit still and allow my mind to quiet fairly well; however the arm flapping and mouth breathing came as a surprise. How could I quiet my mind with all of that movement and counting?

It blew my theory that meditation needed to be calm

and relaxing. I googled Gurmukh and looked over her website. She seemed vaguely familiar. I remembered buying a prenatal yoga DVD over five years earlier, pregnant with Michael. I had struggled to keep up to the energetic teacher. I perused Gurmukh's collection of DVDs for sale on her site. The prenatal DVD was indeed among them.

I recalled her melodic, nurturing tone describing the exercises then saying, "okay, go," as she flapped her arms repeatedly for what felt like hours, encouraging, "keep up!" A likeable, light-hearted woman with radiant skin and an equal dose of wisdom and humour in her teachings, Gurmukh was the Richard Simmons of the kundalini world. She kicked my butt, pregnant and not.

I didn't know the difference between styles of yoga. Gurmukh shared kundalini yoga. The meditation she forwarded was a *kriya*[1]: a tool for achieving focus, disciplining the mind and connecting mind, body, spirit and Source.

I googled the opening chant. I had no idea how to pronounce or execute it. The first video I found featured a man in a loin cloth, seated on a wood floor, belting out the chant in a forced, deep voice, too boisterous for my comfort. The next starred a girl in a flowing top and head scarf, seated on the grass in a park — more my pace. Until she spoke with a thick Polish accent, complicating the Sanskrit pronunciation. *Next.*

I reenacted a version of *The Three Bears* — not too hot, not too cold — and reviewed several videos to ensure a consensus among sources before I chose a style. I practiced the words along with the video. *Ong Namo Guru Dev Namo:* the opening chant, spoken aloud three times, created the sacred space for my kriya practice.

Cross-legged on the floor, hands in prayer position at my

heart, eyes closed, I drew a deep inhalation, paused, then in a low, steady tone, slowly chanted, "Oooooooooooooong Naaamooooooooooo Guru Deeeeeeeeeev Naaaamoooooooooooo," three times. The sound of my voice vibrated through my heart and out through my thumbs pressed against my sternum. I inhaled and paused, my scalp and shoulder blades tingled. The air felt buzzed around me. I dropped my hands from my heart to my belly and parted my palms. I began the *Breath of Ten*. It commanded all of my focus to count, breathe and move my arms while keeping the rest of my body and mind still.

I called Anna after practice to compare notes and learn about her personal kriya.

"I got Breath of Ten, Steph." Out of our group, we were the only two with a shared kriya. "It's so weird. But I feel so focused after."

"I know what you mean," I agreed. "It's so much easier to sit in meditation after the kriya. It's like it lingers after practice."

Years earlier, in my fitness regimen, I preferred high intensity interval training. The method maximized my allotted workout time, challenged my cardiovascular level and allowed the work to continue after my session finished. For me, Breath of Ten was the yoga equivalent of high intensity interval training. No wonder Gurmukh looked so robust.

After a few days the practice felt less complicated. I found a rhythm between the movements and the breathing which allowed me to sink deeper into the kriya. The whole process flowed from opening mantra to closing movements. I had ninety days to get through Breath of Ten. It never occurred to me that Breath of Ten was needed to get me through the next ninety days.

27

NATURE SMELLS

Ten of us met at the trailhead. We hiked Two Pine in pairs as part of Alora's regular Thursday evening yoga class. We arrived at the top at seven-thirty and spread our yoga mats over wild grass. I tried not to crush the violet vetch that wrapped itself around the edge of my mat.

Alora led a reflective practice. I balanced on one leg, knee bent, arms wound around each other like twisting branches: eagle's pose. I gazed at the mountains, not far in the distance, sun on my face, sensing the quiet focus and power of the great bird perched on the hilltop. Wind had commanded the entire day, as can happen in the foothills, but was less powerful during our gathering — forceful enough to keep the mosquitoes at bay yet not blow us off the peak.

"Feel your place in nature," guided Alora. "Feel yourself expand into the surroundings and join seamlessly with your environment, one with nature."

I breathed deeply, inviting the place where I ended and the air began, to merge. I felt no end to me, no skin, no form.

I imagined the wind blowing through me. In that moment the air held its breath — deafening silence.

The wind suddenly stopped completely. The stillness consumed my attention as my environment consumed me. No longer an observer of the wind, I felt a part of it. Inside of it, perhaps, or it inside of me.

We stepped out of the posture. The wind exhaled: a hurricane after the stillness. The trees chatted non-stop, the long grasses took turns playing each other like violin strings.

"Bring your hands together at the heart in lotus flower *mudra*."

At first we formed the bud, then extended our fingers slowly, allowing the flower to bloom out of our hands.

"Now raise your blossoming lotus overhead and offer it skyward."

The aroma of wild flowers overpowered me. A whiff of wild roses had caught my nose on our hike up but at that moment it was as if I could smell the cumulative fragrance of *every* flower on the hill. As if, in my silent reverence and receptive state, amplified by the collective state of the group, the flora reached out to me as I reached my blossom over-head. I gorged on their aliveness, unsure how long their intoxicating synergy would ride the breeze.

We completed our practice with many moments of unimposed silence. I began to understand the difference between a stretch of silence and moments. A stretch put a timeline on my practice: the eleven minutes of clock-peek-ing. Many moments strung together when time left the equation and I simply slipped into each moment as it surfaced like soap bubbles from a child's wand.

I sank into the silence, the summer sun setting over the mountains and another gift of a day coming to a close. The silence had become a warm blanket, a departure from how it felt the last time I stood on the mountain top. I craved it, relished it, longed for it and bathed in it. My senses came alive in it, and once engaged, the heightened sensory experience flowed throughout my day, enhancing the taste of food, the smell of the air, the drumbeat of music, the song of birds, and the feeling of the earth under my feet. My mind didn't chatter. There was no room: the silence full with awareness.

On the walk down the mountain, I casually mentioned both events I had noticed during our practice to Louise, ready to change the subject if she looked at me strangely.

"I had that *exact* same experience with the overwhelming flower fragrance during lotus mudra. I was struck by the timing."

So it wasn't just me.

I lay in bed that night still electrified by the evening's practice. The events teased a memory from the recesses of my mind. Another day in nature, during my life in Banff, made its way to the front of my thoughts.

My roommate at the time was from Quebec. She spoke fluent English but sometimes melded her English with French, which always made me chuckle because she never noticed.

"Can you pass me the can of pêche?"

It was a good thing I spoke French.

We took off on a bike trip one day. We packed a lunch and headed to Canmore on our mountain bikes: the wrong equipment for the job. This was long before the paved Legacy Trail that cyclists now enjoy, safe from highway tourist traffic and semis hauling gasoline or groceries. We slogged along the shoulder of the highway, sucking in car exhaust.

We made it to Canmore and continued along the river

through the townsite and up the mountain base to the Nordic Center for a bathroom break. We climbed back in the saddle and followed the Banff Trail mountain bike track through the heavily-forested mountainside. Navigating rocks, roots and stumps kept our reflexes alert.

We pulled our bikes into the trees, off the track, and sat on the spongy earth for a long-awaited lunch break. I had eaten barely half my sandwich when we heard it. Like the snort of a horse. Only we knew it wasn't a horse.

We didn't leach time to confirm what our senses and the hair on our arms knew. Bear. Run! I tossed my sandwich into my pack and my pack over one shoulder while climbing into the peddles. My legs had never moved so fast. It wasn't until the trail spit us out at the Banff Springs Golf Course that we slowed our spin. Then nervous laughter consumed us in an effort to escort the adrenaline from our spent bodies.

I returned to the apartment to discover three messages on our answering machine. "It's your mother, call me."

"Your mother again, want to know how your ride went."

"Still your mother, let me know you're safe."

I don't know that I told her about the bear. Probably best not to increase her cause for concern. Or maybe I did, because those kind of stories had to be told.

I chuckled in bed at the memory. Life in Banff. I could say that Mother Nature sharpened my senses, but it was more than that. It was as if she delivered them to me.

28

DARK SECRETS

"*The breezes at dawn have secrets to tell you. Don't go back to sleep! You must ask for what you really want. Don't go back to sleep! People are going back and forth across the doorsill where the two worlds touch, the door is round and open. Don't go back to sleep!*" The writings of the thirteenth century mystic poet, Rumi, crossed my path several times from a variety of sources. The words called to me, as he called to me, again and again, begging my attention.

With the kids on summer break, and no need for routine, I struggled to feel energized in the third chakra phase of our year. It was a departure from the explosive, endless energy I had felt at the retreat. I stayed in bed as long as I could in the mornings, not the norm for me, especially with at least one of the kids usually up before six.

Odd occurrences repeatedly woke me in the early morning hours: the birds, my cat, Steve's bathroom breaks, the train. It was non-stop. One thing each and every morning would wake me. And every morning, I would struggle to go back to sleep, and end up dragging myself out of bed several hours later.

What would happen if I got up when I was woken? Was there a message for me in the early morning hours? Had the poet discovered magic in those hours? *Okay, I'll get up as soon as I wake. Well, ... as long as it's after five.* With two young children, the days were long enough. If there was one season in Western Canada to wake early though, it was summer. I wouldn't be at risk of freezing and the sun would be up by six — no better time of year to find out if there was purpose in those hours.

The caw of a crow entered my dream. It took time before it actually woke me. I opened my eyes. *Okay, this is it.* It was five-fifty. He had been cawing nonstop for some time. *If I get up and he stops, then he was meant to wake me.*

As soon as my feet hit the floor, the cawing stopped. My wake-up call. My Mother Nature alarm clock. I answered immediately by crawling back into bed and sleeping until seven.

I was up. Why did I crawl back into bed? I tried not to internalize it but I was upset with myself for not following my plan to see the early-wake-up-thing through. To get up, go for a walk, watch the sunrise, meditate, be in nature, whatever, something, anything but remain in bed.

I called Anna later and shared my disappointment.

"You, of all people," she responded, "should take advantage of the time to sleep. After so many years of sleepless nights you have some serious sleep hours to bank."

Bye bye birdie.

The following morning a robin's song greeted me. She sang so loud I got up to see if I had left the window open. It was hot. I looked at the clock: exactly five o'clock. As soon as I got to the window, she stopped. *Just one time. I can make tea and sack out in front of cartoons with the kids later if I'm too tired to get through the afternoon.*

I slipped on my housecoat and crept to the lower level of the house. Stepping out onto the patio, I sat down in one of the two deck chairs. My head was fuzzy and I had to squint through one eye at a time, not ready to open together. I couldn't stop yawning. The sky was dark — not the pitch black of night — more the deep blue of the sea. The air was still and I could not see much around me. The chair faced south and I stared off at the sparse parade of headlights on the highway across the valley in the distance.

It was quiet on my patio and even though the air was still, there was an interesting quality to it: a fullness, a density I hadn't noticed before. It was as if the space around me was heavier than usual, insulating me. There was a sound as well, a tone to the heaviness that I could hear — not quite a hum — higher pitched and constant. Different from how it sounded to be outdoors any other time of day. It could have been the quiet and the darkness that allowed my senses to receive more information.

I closed my eyes and drifted into a peaceful meditation, allowing my mind to clear and my body to settle. It was harder to keep a clear head since I was searching for what existed in the early morning hours. I was on a mission and I feared that if I couldn't settle myself, I might miss it, not knowing what *it* was. I had pried myself out of my warm, comfy bed and, damn it, I was going to get to the bottom of this early morning mystery.

I sat in the stillness, eyes closed, listening: birds, the cars in the distance, the air conditioning units of my neighbours switching on and off. I wondered what it would sound like if I lived in the country instead of the city. Pure nature, no whirring fans and hot tub heaters.

I don't know how long I sat with my eyes closed, but when I opened them, I could make out shapes of shrubs in my garden and the chain link fence behind them. I sat, still, as more images emerged from the fading darkness. The sky glowed with a strange light that seeped in from nowhere to brighten the entire sky, one shade of blue at a time. Every moment birthed more light.

Soothing blues turned to purple, pink then soft orange as the mountaintops in the distance took on a warm glow. The entire range became bathed in pink, orange and gold. My wind chimes started to dance and sing as the air began to move with the rise of the sun, as if Mother Earth was taking her first breath of the day. The temperature dropped as she inhaled.

My neighbour's kitchen light flicked on, distracting, but not enough to lure my gaze from the amber mountains. I could hear my children running about the house. Steve would be getting ready for work. I breathed deeply, waking my body from its comfortable position on the chair.

I stood up, stretched my arms overhead and felt all my muscles engage and then release as I exhaled my arms down and turned my gaze back to the mountains. Bright yellow sunlight illuminated their faces and moved quickly across the foothills in front of them like a wildfire spreading down the mountains and across the fields.

"Thank you," I whispered, and I welcomed the sun and the day ahead. As I turned to go inside, I suddenly remembered the reason I had come to the patio in the first place. I wondered if the early waking experiment had revealed its purpose to me.

It was worth the waking. Yes. The day would be filled with blue skies, wispy clouds and prominent mountains in the distance, but only in the early morning hours would I see the steady giants glow and dance in the sun's light, welcoming the day.

I had always loved sunsets and found myself each day facing west to the mountains, drawn into the peaceful beauty and the sorrowful departure of the setting sun. It was different than in the early morning. People were still awake and active at sunset. Children played in the park and adults barbecued on their decks. I lived east of the mountains, in their foothills, and the sun set behind them.

Only in the light of the rising sun could I see their faces filled with colour. I had seen Mother Earth get ready for sleep many times. To watch her wake and take her first full breath of the day was pure magic. In his poem, Rumi may have written about night and day colliding, or the physical world and the spiritual, but that morning, I felt the "*two worlds*" he wrote of were mine and hers.

After prying myself from bed at the robin's call, I was done telling the story of sleep deprivation to myself. I was tired, not from lack of sleep but from holding onto the resentment of getting up so often with the kids and sacrificing the energy I once had. The simple act of letting it go restored vitality to my body and my spirit. I dropped my expectations around sleep.

I accepted it as an opportunity to capture a dream before it disintegrated back to where it came from; to be private audience to the full blue moon moments before it dropped over the Rockies in the wee hours; to catch Venus dancing with crescent moon in the glow of winter snow as a shooting star skated by; to scribe the details of a dreamtime story. All of it a gift. I no longer felt tired. I felt wide awake.

29

DIE IN THE FIRE OR RISE LIKE THE PHOENIX

I booked an appointment with Karen, since our paths continued to cross. She was a medium, as well as a Shaman, and I wished to add a reading with her to my list of experiences. I was devouring all things mystical and controversial with a voracious appetite.

Ever since the fire ceremony where the wind caused the hairs on the back of my neck to stand, I wanted to meet with Karen one-on-one. I felt she may have some answers for me. I had not been to a medium before. A palm reader, yes; tea leaf reader, yes; clairvoyant, yes. I was a lover of the mystical and had buried it along with the hidden treasure of purpose when the lure and responsibilities of adult life took over.

Karen greeted me at the door to her home with a hug and led me to her client room in the basement. I sat opposite her.

"How do I know what my purpose is?" I asked.

"You're struggling," she replied. "You're stuck. When you become unstuck the world will open up to you."

She kept saying, "you being you ..." What did she mean by that? It was as if she knew who I was but I didn't know who I was. Who was I? That's what *I* was trying to figure out. Did she know something I didn't? Why didn't I ask her to clarify? She spoke to me like I should understand exactly what she meant. I didn't. But I didn't want to let on that I didn't. Talk about futility. No wonder I didn't know who I was. I was afraid to ask.

She suggested I conduct a fire ceremony on my own to release the issue. She handed me her book. It outlined the process for releasing such issues by breaking contracts that had been made by one of my ancestors or me — in this or a past lifetime. These contracts could take the form of running themes in my life: limitations and barriers, health issues or repeated behaviours. I thanked her and returned home. I took her advice: "Shaman says why not today," and went straight to work with the fire.

I followed the steps for the fire ceremony. I clearly identified the issue of knowing my purpose in this life and offered it up exactly as outlined in Karen's book. My first personal fire ceremony went well.

The next day, my world crashed. Turmoil in the house almost caused us to cancel the family vacation. Old behaviour patterns with Steve, patterns that I thought I had left behind, resurfaced. Issues buried deep emerged. I criticized him. He blamed me. Voices raised. Tears burst. Crap spilled out like an overflowing toilet all over our morning holiday packing.

Karen's book warned about fallout after a release, but I felt as if I'd taken ten steps backward. My spiritually-awakened high disappeared and my connection to magic snapped. The whole damn process was broken. I searched for it, desperately trying to reconnect.

We continued with the holiday, for the sake of the kids, departing several hours later than planned. I felt sick to my stomach and emotionally exhausted as we drove through the mountains, arriving at the resort after dark.

I fumbled for my Zen. I sat on a peaceful deck attached to a four-star hotel room, surrounded by nature, on the top of a mountain in the middle of the Rockies. Peace eluded me. I spent the time replaying the fire ceremony. Had I asked for the wrong thing? Had I released something I thought I understood but maybe didn't? Had I worded it wrong?

Alora had requested we revisit our first three chakras prior to the next gathering, in order to move from our foundation to the higher chakras. I hadn't done that. Actually, I'd been remiss in doing the exercises that accompanied each chakra from the book Alora assigned us at the start of the year: *Chakra Balancing* by Anodea Judith. Coincidentally, I had brought my workbook with me on our family holiday. After deciding that sitting and staring at the mountains in a meditative stupor proved fruitless, I opened my book and began working through the writing exercises.

I wrote my answers to the second chakra questions. *My weaknesses are: feeling guilty regarding balance of time/energy between kids, hubby, me and work.* I knew I hadn't resolved that issue, that I may never, but I needed to revisit it before I could move on. Even acknowledging it in writing on the page, somehow allowed me to accept it as a part of my journey. I reconfirmed my commitment to second chakra practice and to dance, play and be creative with the kids, as well as make intimacy with Steve a regular practice. The last one felt nearly impossible since we were now barely speaking to each other and even avoiding eye contact.

I began immediately with the kids — playing mini-golf and swimming. I was fortunate to be in the mountains surrounded by the healing energy of nature during an explosive time. We managed to salvage the family holiday, even extending it by a day, but the tension between Steve and me remained.

The kids slept in the backseat of the car on the drive home. The fire between my husband and me continued to simmer beneath the surface. No solution presented itself, no sign of peace or middle ground appeared. Defensive remarks and cold shoulders were all that remained. He finally threw out the D word, something I had done several times before in exasperation. For *him* to consider divorce, I knew the situation was dire and not much appeared evident for salvage. In that moment, however, I felt relief. But not about the prospect of separating.

My relief came from the fact that we were finally *both* frustrated enough to make a change. Years of sleeplessness, poor communication, resentment and emotional withdrawal were not going to be erased overnight. I didn't know how we would suddenly heal from years of relationship damage, but at least I knew we were both fed up with the status quo. He wanted better. And I did too: something honest and easy and joyful. A life where everyone felt comfortable being themselves, expressing their own needs and desires; where the people in our family felt not only supported but nourished, encouraged and deeply loved; where we cheered for one another and became each other's biggest fans.

If the fire release was the catalyst for the sobering realization that I had to get honest about who I was, where I was, and where I wanted to be, then it proved a powerful practice. I couldn't dress this up, apply essential oils and a couple gemstones and call it a day. All I could do was clean up my shit.

There were no more defences, no illusions and no more

gloss. The remainder of the drive home echoed silence. Not the intentional silence of meditation, but an exhausted, depleted silence that resulted from the ravaging fire of third chakra. The forest had been stripped of its foliage.

Once home, I connected with my yoga community via email. We had not come together in a long time, but the emails kept us in touch and provided support. I had made some decisions on the drive back from holidays. I needed to allow Steve the space to make his own decisions, while I got clear on mine.

I shared with Alora and the group how I reviewed our workbook to realize my foundation needed reinforcement. I may have, in my excitement and awe of what was waking up inside me, begun to lay down new foundation without first removing the old. I had simply placed fresh footings on a rotting structure.

I clicked away at the keyboard, informing the group of my decision to leave real estate. I cancelled my license before our fourth chakra gathering. I needed to eject things from my life that no longer worked, that drained my energy, drew my attention from what needed it most: my family. The roles of Realtor, personal trainer, mom, wife, and the torrid (although invigorating) pace of awakening, were wearing away at my family's foundation.

The summer's heat had produced many fires and, although scorched, I felt strangely strengthened by it all. Tender and raw, I no longer feared the flames, although I had much healing to do and no idea how it would happen or how long it would take.

"What is to give light must first endure burning."
~Victor Frankl

PART V

HEART CHAKRA

HEAL

All that healing requires
is a gentle touch.

30

A SMILING HEART

I had the packing of my yoga bag down to a science. I tossed it, and another bag with nightgown and personal essentials, into the car and drove to the lodge. I planned to stay at Sacred Forest the evening before the fourth chakra gathering. I placed my gear in the red room, made myself a tea, and melted into the couch. Only three of us lounged around for the evening and retired early. I slept like a baby — not one of my babies, mind you. Once asleep, I didn't stir until morning.

I woke early, listening for sounds of life in the cabin. I heard nothing. I slipped on my yoga pants and sweater, grabbed a blanket off the couch in the living room, and snuck through the sunroom to the back porch overlooking the pasture. I took up position on the large stump and wrapped myself in the blanket and the comfort of silence and nature.

I sat motionless on the stump, allowing nature to restore me. My numb state helped me slip into meditation and quiet reflection. I had come to know the healing nature and peace of early morning, the simplicity before sunrise. I remained in my blanketed cocoon until noise inside the cabin alerted me to the arrival of others. I left my perch and headed back inside. In the kitchen, Alora set out oranges and Anna boiled water for tea.

In a steady stream of arrivals, the group gathered once again, this time to investigate and celebrate fourth chakra — heart chakra or *anahata*, Sanskrit for *unbeaten* or *unstruck*. I embraced the return to the lodge, the group, and the movement forward into fourth chakra discovery. Autumn loomed: my favourite season. The sun's rays still heated the mid-day while the early mornings and late evenings shifted to cooler, refreshing air, a welcome reprieve from the intensity of the summer's heat.

I sipped my tea in the sunroom while Alora and the others unpacked their mats and settled in. As I twisted my torso from side to side, stretching my body, I noticed something bizarre. I realized the pain in my spine had shifted with each chakra. It had originated at the base of my spine, referring down the backs of my legs, when I began the year in yoga. I suddenly remembered that days before second chakra gathering, the pain left my lower spine and locked up my back across the hips.

An acute attack of pain in the low spine and legs surfaced during fire retreat, when we revisited the lower chakras. That pain quickly resolved after the retreat and my mid back began causing problems while the lower spine and legs felt better than ever. Sitting on my mat, tea in hand, I twisted to one side, then the other. My mid back was free of pain, but stiffness seized my back at the level of my bra strap, behind my heart. Tightness between the shoulder blades prohibited me from deepening the movement.

I recalled the first meeting of the year, when Alora briefly mentioned kundalini, asking to let her know if the energy was moving too quickly for anyone, she would hook us up with someone who could help. I didn't understand what she had been referring to that first day, so I dismissed it. Her words returned as I contemplated my experience with what she had described: kundalini energy moving up my spine.

I felt fine, other than shifting physical discomfort, which remained tolerable. I saw no need to inform her or seek assistance with the issue, which I knew would shift again toward the end of heart chakra inquiry. *What happens when it runs out of spine? When it reaches the chakras in the head? Forty days of bad hair?*

The others settled into their spots in the sunroom and we shared our experiences of the long third chakra summer while we finished our tea.

"Create a list of people you need to forgive in your life," Alora instructed.

We began our yoga with our journals. I wrote the word forgiveness on the left side of the page and underlined it. At the top of the list I wrote: *me.*

After all the inquiry and discovery, I understood that I was my toughest critic. That I was hardest on myself and was the cause of my struggle. I needed to forgive myself for choices I had made and reactions to the choices of others. I needed to not dwell on the details. I couldn't dredge up the bad relationships — neither my parents' divorce, nor my first husband's and mine. It felt fruitless to haul out every argument, revisit wrongs or berate bad choices. I needed simply to forgive all, in one fell swoop. Exhausted and depleted, my days of struggle and fire were over. It was time to be kind to myself.

I wrote more names on the list of people to forgive, obvious ones. Steve's name, of course. I placed it directly under mine. I needed to forgive him so we could move forward. And I allowed myself to do something I hadn't in a long time, something I considered dealt with long ago. I added the name of my biological father.

I thought I'd come to terms with those early memories. Repressed emotions ran deep. I thought I'd talked it out enough in my head over the years. It was time to stop letting the first five years of my life dictate the following thirty. Sometimes a story just needs to stop being told.

We moved into our physical practice. Sitting on our mats, eyes closed, hands folded in our laps or resting on our legs, we drew attention to our breath.

"Inhale a silent *aham*," said Alora, "and exhale a silent *prema* ... I am divine love."

Aham, I inhaled, prema, I exhaled. I sank into my body, my breath, the mantra and the familiar sanctuary of the sunroom. Aham prema.

"Release the mantra and come to standing," said Alora. "Bring to mind thoughts to smile-up your heart. Think of what makes you happiest and envision your heart growing an enormous grin with the memory of your happy thoughts."

It was easy to put the dark memories aside because there were many beautiful memories to conjure. I directed my memories to my teens and of sitting in front of the barn with my mom, aunts and cousins watching the new litter of kittens play and chase each other around while the snow slowly receded in the warm spring sun. I recalled happy memories to smile-up my heart. There were many: cuddling the kids as they slept in my arms; their smiles and laughs; how they light up at the sight of Mom; our Maui wedding, on the beach, toes in sand, ocean waves prompting us to speak our vows louder as they bounded noisily in celebration onto the surrounding lava rocks. I recalled playing cards with Steve on the deck of our condo in Kauai by candlelight as the scent of plumeria wafted on the island breeze. I smiled. My heart smiled.

In our happy state, Alora led us through a series of gratitude sun salutations. Beginning in mountain pose at the top of our mats, we formed a blossom with our hands pressed together, fingertips touching. Slowly we raised our hands up in front of us, gradually opening the blossom, allowing our middle fingers to part first, followed by second and fourth, the petals of the lotus, leaving pinkies and thumbs connected. We held the full bloom overhead, offering it as gratitude to someone in our lives. No details required, we simply held a vision of that person clearly in our mind. If we began to struggle at any time, we smiled-up our hearts with warm memories and resumed the practice.

I raised my first bloom to Steve. I opened my hands and released the offering to the sky. I swept my hands down to my mat as I folded forward and then stepped back to plank and flowed: upward dog, downward dog, stepping back up to the top of my mat to rest in mountain pose. I held the image of Steve through the full sun salutation. Another bloom, this time for Michael, followed by one for Khali, family members, friends and, finally, a long indulgent sun salutation dedicated to me completed my gratitude practice. We moved into heart-chakra-focused yoga asanas, bending back into camel pose, hearts lifted to the ceiling, opening our chests in bow pose and peeling our upper bodies off the mat in cobra.

Alora read out the affirmations and we repeated them in the poses.

"I love myself for who I am and the potential within me. All past hurt I release into the hands of love. I am grateful for all the love in my life. Others love the best they can. If someone doesn't love me *enough* they may be limited in their expression of love and deserve my compassion."

My breath caught in my collarbones as I arched into the poses. I had noticed for some time that my breathing felt restricted. I only realized it through my asana practice when I slowed down and focused on breath and movement. When I tried to take a deep breath, it felt as though I could only fill the top half of my lungs, my shoulders rising as I tried to draw in more air. I strained to expand yet couldn't make progress even with the yoga and breathing exercises. It had become more pronounced as my practice deepened and my meditations required fuller breath and longer periods of holding. No matter how I tried, I could not expand the flow of air in my body.

We sat on our mats as Alora shared the meditation practice for fourth chakra: *Metta Bhavana*, the cultivation of loving kindness. First we warmed our hearts again, invoking the smile. We closed our eyes and repeated after Alora:

"May I live in safety, be happy, be healthy, live with ease. May I dance freely in love."

She instructed us to call someone we cared deeply for to mind — a spouse, child, parent, dear friend — and hold them in our minds and hearts while we repeated the phrase." May you live in safety, be happy, be healthy, live with ease. May you dance freely in love."

Alora asked us to bring to mind a neutral person — a child's teacher, a clerk at a grocery store, someone we encountered in our day but didn't know well. Once again, we repeated the practice, directing the blessing toward them, holding a vision of them in our hearts and minds. I directed the practice toward a neighbour of mine. It felt good to wish kind thoughts for someone else and not have them know, eliminating the ego's need for recognition.

I sat, content on my mat, as Alora asked us to bring to mind someone who needed help, someone with whom we struggled. She reminded us to smile-up our hearts as we held the image of the person in our hearts and minds, to stay in a place of love as we repeated: "May you live in safety, be happy, be healthy, live with ease. May you dance freely in love."

I had to smile-up my heart a couple times before I felt enough warmth to repeat the phrase. The details of my less-than-ideal relationship with the person forced the warmth to dissipate from my heart. It required disciplined retrieval of the smiley heart to continue to offer a blessing to someone with whom I struggled.

Alora told us to choose a phrase for our home practice of Metta Bhavana and make it personal, using words that came naturally to us. Not much of the exercise felt natural.

Lying on my back in savasana, I thought about how I once felt so full of love in my life, with so much love to give to everyone. Supine on my mat in that moment, however, I felt depleted. I realized love is like food: I eat to nourish myself. If I don't eat, my body robs from itself in order to continue functioning, depleting its resources.

I saw love the same way. Only I expected others to love me enough to fill me up, which is like needing others to feed me and then feeling resentful in my depleted state that they left me to starve. Others weren't responsible for feeding me. Once old enough to feed myself, I became responsible for my own nourishment, my own refuelling. I made conscious, healthy and intelligent choices about the foods I put in my body yet made little effort to love myself.

A snore broke my thoughts, more like a snort — Britt

perhaps. I went back to my breath and my contemplation of self-love. I saw a flight attendant, standing at the front of the airplane, poised in preflight presentation, oxygen mask in hand, as the prerecorded audio instructed those travelling with small children, or others requiring assistance, to secure their own mask first before placing one on someone else.

I had been busy placing masks on everyone *but* myself, which hadn't taken that much of a toll, until I had kids and mask-placing became a twenty-four-hour job. Prior to that, I had tried to place masks on the men in my life, looking for someone to place one on me. All those years, I'd missed a crucial step: securing the mask on myself first.

31

THROUGH THE EYES OF A CHILD

Our guest presenter arrived: a man who specialized in chiropractic care with a transformational approach. He worked to help people function on a higher level of physical and spiritual wellness. I admit I don't remember much of the session. I must have been in la la land or still blissed out by one too many of Alora's chocolate bliss balls.

Some parts of our journey grabbed me more than others but I found, even in the less-memorable experiences, a drop of nectar always presented itself. The drop I received from the presenter that afternoon was when he spoke about transformation:

"Once you start to shift," he said, "you no longer have the same physical body."

His words stunned me. Prior to fourth chakra gathering, I had experienced several days of headaches — out of character for me. I had booked an eye exam, years overdue, to see if I needed a new prescription for glasses. I never wore mine, which I'd had since I was a teenager. I was nearsighted and my night vision sucked. I resolved to not even try to read road signs or the hanging menu boards in fast food restaurants until I was directly underneath them. I played a lot of sports and repeatedly putting my glasses on and taking them off gave me headaches as a girl, so I decided to make do with my limited vision and spent my life with my glasses securely in their case in my purse. I pulled them out to watch live hockey games, theatre and special performances, to see the expressions on the actors' faces or numbers on the hockey jerseys.

As I headed to the optometrist, I considered treating myself to a stylish set of frames and actually wearing my glasses. I was scared something more serious might be wrong with my eyes. The eye doc performed a range of exams, including what seemed like a particularly long vision chart session.

He pushed the equipment away from my face and his chair back from mine. "Your vision tested 20/10. In twenty years of practice, I've seen that result maybe three or four times, and always in children."

What was interesting about the whole eyesight issue, was that I clearly remembered wanting glasses as a kid because other kids had them. I'm not entirely sure I needed them then, but as my teenage years went by, my eyes seemed to oblige and provided the desired outcome. Sometime during my yoga journey, clarity had returned to my vision.

We grabbed blankets and headed outside with Alora for one final meditation of the day. We walked across the property, past the wood shop, the chicken coops, the equipment shed, and through the gates to the horse pasture.

I shared a corner of a blanket with Anna, and chased the creepy crawlies from our fabric real estate. The horses stood near us most of the meditation. The constant trickle of the creek hypnotized me. My gaze gently fixed on the other side of the water where the tall, thick evergreens stood: the healing green of heart chakra.

"Anahata's element is air," began Alora. "Breathe in the energy of heart chakra. Breathe in the green of the trees. This chakra is our centre of love and self-love. Healing begins with heart chakra."

I felt my breath flow in and out. I focused my attention on my heart. My chest grew warmer with each breath.

Back at the cabin, we selected our beads for heart chakra: rose quartz. Infusing the soft pink stones with blessings proved easy. Not easy emotionally, but the places that needed healing and love in my life were clear. The people who needed forgiveness and compassion were just as clear. I slipped into the silent craft as I slipped each bead on the string.

Heart chakra colours include the pink rose quartz and the healing green of nature. Heart chakra also rules the lungs. Sadness, grief, heartache, and loneliness are issues of *anahata* chakra. Love, compassion, self-love, forgiveness, and generosity: all antidotes.

We completed our practice with enough time for one last tribute to heart chakra. Alora asked us to partner up and practice the art of giving and receiving as we traded hand and foot massages with each other. Anna and I paired up for the decadent treat. It felt odd having my best friend rub my feet, but I surrendered to her nurturing touch and felt grateful for the caring attention. When it came time for me to reciprocate, I enjoyed giving as much as I had enjoyed receiving.

The day felt easy, almost mundane. No striking, fleeting

moments of awe followed by desperate attempts to cling to those moments. The chatter in my head remained minimal. I'm not sure if third chakra was simply a hard one to top, or if I really was coming into my own spiritual practice. I believe the fires of summer had burned up much of what I had long stored away. I was finally receptive to healing.

32

FINDING HEALING CLOSE TO HOME

I sat on a park bench at a playground near my home, hoping to practice Metta Bhavana and reflect in nature while the kids played. One of the neighbourhood moms sat down beside me. I knew her only casually, a friendly lady, in the midst of surviving — and thriving through — breast cancer. She operated a day home, even while undergoing treatments, and brought her wards to the park to play.

"You know, I'm doing very well but I could use some exercising. The medications put on much of the weight." She'd come to Canada from Iran. Her first Canadian home was Montreal. She went from speaking only Iranian to learning French, then she moved to Calgary and added English. My plan had been side-tracked. I realized she needed to share and that giving her my attention and the information she sought about exercise was more important than my meditation.

"Have you considered complementary alternative therapies like Reiki?" I asked her.

"Ah, yes, I go to Sophie."

"Who?" I asked.

"You do not know Sophie? Ah! She is Reiki master. Gives beautiful treatments. Only a few houses away. Just there. You stay here and watch children while I go and get her number for you."

The lady she spoke of lived almost directly behind me.

"Her fee is very good," She said when she'd returned, handing me a piece of paper with Sophie's number. "You go. You will love her."

I realized my arrogance and ignorance. I was not in the park that day to share my knowledge with her. She had just shared hers with me — an unexpected gift for which I thanked her. It had been difficult for me to find the time and justify the expense for the regular Reiki treatments I had grown to love at the wellness center nearby. I immediately booked my first treatment with the Reiki neighbour.

SOPHIE OPENED HER FRONT DOOR. The inviting aroma of essential oils wafted through the doorway. There was an equally inviting expression on her face and in her voice. "Hellooo," she greeted me in a melodic French accent. Her dark hair was pulled off her face and clipped up in a loose bun in back. Her round face beamed kindness which put me at ease and in good hands.

Vibrant pieces of Middle Eastern art adorned her entry. Enlarged pictures of three beautiful children hung on the walls. Sophie led me into her treatment room, the main floor den. Her Reiki table stood in the centre, a large bookshelf against one wall, a wooden desk against the other and there was a window opposite the door.

I hopped up on the treatment table, quickly scanning

the selection on the bookshelves: books on healing, Reiki, chakras and meditation. A diffuser intermittently puffed essential oils into the air: earthy, yet sweet. Candles glowed on the desk, their light animating the faces of stone angels.

"We moved to Canada from Dubai. It was a bit of a shock, especially the winter, but my children are making good friends here. Now ... what is happening with you?"

I mentioned my participation in the year in yoga and the new experiences unfolding around me.

"Lie down." She scanned my body with her hands.

"Your body is divided in half, split at heart chakra. Energy's not moving between your upper and lower body." She slowly moved her hands across my body. She looked as though she was listening to something. "Hmm, you want to take in as much of this new journey as possible and detach from the rest of your daily routine, yes?"

She wasn't wrong about me wanting to detach. I craved immersion in the yoga, meditations, mantras and all that made me feel light and joyful. The daily grind of dishes, dinners and laundry held little appeal. I wanted to claim every moment in my day to further my exploration. My initial satisfaction in finding yoga in boiling eggs — in the daily details of life — had turned into an intense drive for deeper spiritual experience.

"You need to ground deeply," she continued. "Spend time playing on the floor with your children, time in nature with them. Separate your time in spiritual things. Keep your practice and meditations sacred, not interfering in life with family. It will all come together, but it doesn't have to be all at once."

I didn't want to separate the two. I wanted to blend sacred with family. I didn't want two lives, I wanted one whole life. Unfortunately, the scale had tipped along the way and self-exploration consumed my attention.

Chanting during most of the session, Sophie practiced *Karuna* Reiki on me. Karuna is Sanskrit, meaning *compassionate action*. It was fascinating how the two different traditions, Sanskrit and Japanese, blended together in my treatment. Sensation pulsed through my body as she chanted, different from the electric buzzing I had felt in sessions with my first Reiki practitioner. These were wave-like, moving from my feet upward to my head, strengthening in intensity as we progressed through the session. Pink sheet lightening erupted from behind my closed lids, as though there was an electrical storm inside my body. One wave crested so strong, I thought my head would explode.

I was exhausted after the session. I couldn't put two thoughts together. I felt weightless. Sophie poured me a glass of water and I sipped until I felt able to get off her table and leave.

"You should learn Reiki. It would be very good for you," she said.

"Oh, I don't know. I'm content to receive your lovely treatments. Thank you again."

While I walked the ridge path home, I pondered Sophie's comments about separating the components of my life. Not every moment required inquiry. It was hard to think of doing anything other than yoga, mystical exploration and contemplating the universe. I rejected Sophie's suggestion that at some point I should consider learning Reiki; it didn't feel right to me.

33

ROOM TO BREATHE

I woke the next morning, stretched my arms overhead and took a deep breath. It flowed freely into my lungs, with room to spare, expanding the sides of my ribcage and filling my belly. Instead of my shoulders rising to make room, the air flowed down into generous spaces in my body. It was like taking a breath for the first time.

I stole another and another, certain that at some point my breathing would return to its shallow state. I enjoyed the expansion of my lungs repeatedly throughout the day. I had no idea how long I had been *holding* my breath. My asana practice and my meditations improved. The Reiki session with Sophie had yielded remarkable results.

I chose a yoga DVD to assist with my morning practice, craving variety and challenge. My breath guided my movements instead of being forced by my postures. I inhaled, floating my body upward into position and exhaled, folding and releasing. My new breath persuaded my mind to calm even more.

I reached a new place with my yoga, a place of synergy

with breath and body. I expanded further into each pose with every inhalation and moved deeper into the postures with every exhalation — the union of body, mind and spirit: yoga.

I recalled the seminar on Ayurveda where we practiced the breath-holding exercise. It demonstrated how hard it was to keep something out that wanted to come in and to keep something in that wanted to be let go. The importance of the exercise crystallized once my breath expanded. I had been holding onto much and it was suffocating me. Everything I held took up space, preventing what wanted to flow naturally toward me.

What school didn't teach me, what the workplace couldn't offer me, was what my heart was trying to reveal: I was out of sync, and the way to harmonize was to stop. Stop moving. Stop busying my brain and my life. Stop preoccupying myself with what I thought would be the answer. Stop, and drop everything I was holding onto. Drop it all like the weight and burden it was. Some of it so old, I could hardly believe I had carried it all that way. No wonder my spine had crumbled under the weight.

Put it down. With every exhale, I let go: the busyness, the importance, the pain, the doubt, the victim, the healer, the guilt, the shame, the blame, the security blanket of approval. The emotional dam finally burst and tears flowed with the exhales, pooling on my mat. Some breaths, broken up by sobs, revealed details of the load: my immense expectations of myself and my life.

I needed to be the source of love and value in my life. No man, client, child, certification, achievement, or career could give me what I needed. I needed to forgive myself. Full stop.

Other breaths brought overwhelming relief and release from years of emotional debris. I tried not to grasp at details or force a revisiting of the stories. The flood gates were open wide and I let the water run fast and full. I continued in that way for the duration of my asana practice. My breath flowed, my emotions flowed, my tears flowed and my life began, once again, to flow.

34

AN EARFUL OF ENERGY

Michael had just started kindergarten and already received two time-outs for not listening. He didn't seem to be enjoying the class and I wondered if his ears were bothering him again. We had spent several months with the pediatrician, naturopathic and homeopathic doctors, and craniosacral massage to clear the fluid that had previously gummed up his ears and kept him from hearing. The remedies had proved successful and had helped him avoid the recommended tubes.

I had been seeing Sophie for a while with great success and she had mentioned that I could bring my children to see her. I called to see if she had time for Michael and was able to take him right over. The room, which she usually prepared with candles, angelic statues, aromatherapy and music was, instead, set with Lego, stuffed animals, and a large wooden pirate ship.

Sophie was as attentive with Michael as she'd been with me. It was like having a healer and a child psychologist working with him at the same time. She asked him questions about school and how he enjoyed his teacher and his classmates. She handed me a pen and piece of paper as he checked out the pirate ship and answered her questions.

"I don't know what the teacher wants," he told her. "Not sure what she's asking."

How could you not know? Does she speak in code, another language perhaps? I wanted him to feel safe to share so I didn't intrude on the session or grill him about it later.

Sophie picked up a green crystal, about four or five inches long, and began a stirring motion with the pointy end by his right ear. Preoccupied with Lego at the time, Michael paid no attention to Sophie's movements or treatment other than to answer her gentle questions. She was not actually touching his ear and he couldn't see what she was doing. He stopped playing and began to smile. He leaned toward the crystal like a dog getting scratched behind the ear.

"What are you feeling?" I asked.

"It tickles."

Michael gained immediate relief from his visit with Sophie. When we returned home, I emailed the class volunteer coordinator to schedule a time to volunteer in his class to find out what was going on and how I could help him adjust. Since they were short of volunteers, I got in right away. I had previously found volunteer days at Michael's preschool exhausting, and expected the kindergarten class to leave me equally spent.

Michael introduced me to his class and then they went about their activities while I sat at a table in the back, working on the projects the teacher had assigned me. I paused from my tasks for a moment to be present with the class and the kids. Bright faces beamed from the alphabet carpet, with much energy and enthusiasm. Each wiggly bottom occupied a letter. I sent waves of gratitude to the kids. I envisioned them maintaining their sense of wonder and innocence in the world, spreading it to their families, adults and community — where laughter and play would catch on as quickly as a cold in a kindergarten class.

I listened to the teacher. While the kids sat in front of her, criss-cross applesauce, she outlined their morning, speaking aloud as she arranged items on the Smart Board with her pointer tool.

"First we'll do our carpet time, and then the weather, oops, that's not where that is supposed to go. This needs to move over there ..." Technical difficulties with the board. "Okay, that's better, now the library, we will visit after the weather, oh, that doesn't want to move either."

She spoke in a calm, soft voice as she ran a play by play of her thoughts in concert with the display on the board. I watched Michael fidget and understood his comment to Sophie. At some point in the running dialogue, he tuned his teacher out since he wasn't hearing any clear instructions. It was a matter of communication. Even *I* didn't understand the instructions. With the teacher's energy and style far different from that of his preschool teacher, I was concerned Michael would struggle and continue to get in trouble. *How is this kid going to get through the year?*

Then another thought occurred to me, a different perspective. Although, I had initially disliked the high density of the school of eight-hundred children from kindergarten to grade four, with its accompanying sensory overload, thinking it too much for a kindergartner's tender sensibilities, I had a new thought: *Maybe the large school size is good for Michael and the teacher's style, equally beneficial.*

Maybe he would learn from the environment in ways my impressions and reactions blocked me from considering.

Perhaps Michael would develop focus, patience and listening skills that would help him later. I tried to view the issue as neither good nor bad. Instead of criticizing the teacher or the school, I decided to support his experience as best I could.

I put my heart chakra practices to use and sent gratitude to Michael's teacher, to Michael, the principal, the students, and the community of parents. And I followed that gratitude up with action by volunteering as often as possible to help my son feel comfortable and supported, and to reinforce a strong connection between us. The school year continued to present us with challenges, but I felt part of the solution instead of part of the problem.

35

POURING SALT ON THE WOUND

I called Karen the Shaman for a phone consultation. Since summer holidays, Steve and I had gone about the daily routines of work, and caring for kids and a home. We discussed what each of us needed to be happy, the kind of environment we wished for our home and family, and what we needed from each other. We cleared the air but our relationship remained wounded.

I asked Karen for guidance on healing my relationship with Steve on other levels, since the physical and emotional had been drained. Her instructions were specific. I was to set up a small altar outside. *Where am I going to put that? One, I live in the suburbs; two, my yard is small; and three, my kids play there. Oh, yeah, and I live in Canada.* I had to find things to place on the altar that would survive cold, rain, wind and children. I also needed to find items that held significant representation of Steve, me and Spirit.

I sat on my front lawn with the Buddha statue from my kitchen tucked into my flower bed. I placed a pen to represent me through my new love of journaling, and a golf ball divot repair tool to represent Steve (when you prefer to expedite your shamanic ceremonies like I do, you grab what's handy). I set them next to Buddha, the icon of Spirit. I peered about at the windows of the neighbouring houses. *How crazy do I look? It's not like I'm sacrificing a chicken. It's a simple fire ceremony ... on my lawn ... in the city ... by myself.* Like every other experience in the year in yoga, my inquisitive nature, fascination with the unknown, and dedication to the process, outweighed the awkwardness.

Besides, I loved it — all of it — the intriguing rituals and their origins, the history and ancestry, the rich sensory experiences, and the humour I found in it. I poured an expensive gourmet sea salt circle around us. There we sat, Buddha and me, with the somewhat weather-resistant representatives for Steve and me, and the issue of our relationship, in our salted circle on the grass.

I left the altar on the front lawn for several days, partially hidden by my flower bed. Karen said I would know when it was time to remove it. *How would I know that?* It turned out Mother Nature knew. As I was thinking maybe I should bring Buddha back inside, it started to rain and poured for two days straight. I left Buddha in the rain for cleansing. The downpour stopped after having washed away the salt, and I retrieved the items; I returned Buddha to my kitchen.

A sudden, early snow storm ensued the day after the rains ceased. It was short-lived. When the snow melted, was I surprised to see a perfect circle on my front lawn, like a fairy ring. Dead grass. *Whoops.* In my planning and preparation for the ceremony, I hadn't considered the effect of the salt on the grass.

So much for finding answers to heal my relationship

with Steve. Leaning against the front door, I looked out the window at the perfect circle on the lawn. A voice bubbled up from inside me. *In time, it will grow back naturally and all signs of the damage will be gone.*

36

MR. USUI, I PRESUME?

I took a seat on Sophie's couch, next to a well-dressed woman with white-blonde hair and long, manicured nails. A younger woman with long, lustrous wavy black hair and brilliant eyes sat on the opposite couch. A young man sat on a chair next to the couch. He looked Middle Eastern; I couldn't stop looking at his eyes. I'd never seen such large, dark, compassionate-looking eyes, like the eyes of a doe. He shyly looked away but I was mesmerized and couldn't stop staring.

Sophie prompted our introductions and brief sharings while she poured tea. Her home made the perfect classroom for Reiki: warm, inviting, with essential oils and ginger-verbena tea wafting through the air. I sank into the couch holding my tea. My mother-in-law was looking after the kids at home. Months earlier I would have struggled with getting a babysitter so I could take a day to myself, but I now understood that time spent nourishing me allowed me to better nourish others.

I had been so impressed by the outcome of Michael's session with Sophie, coupled with my own results from her treatments, that I had reconsidered Sophie's suggestion. When she emailed to tell me about the Reiki level 1 group training, I replied, yes. It seemed a natural next step.

Sophie handed a large, white binder to each of us and sat in a chair facing us. She began our lesson with the history of Reiki. Her chair was next to a small round table, more specifically an altar, draped with a silk cloth and set with a large bouquet of coral roses as well as candles, incense and a small brass-framed photo she identified as the founder of Reiki, Mikao Usui.

I followed along in the binder's material. My attention strayed from Sophie's teaching to the photo beneath the roses on her table. I took a heart chakra moment, sending waves of gratitude to Mr. Usui. After all, forty days in heart chakra was predominantly about gratitude and, since I had discovered the sweet, soul-swelling emotion, I wanted to express it everywhere.

Each chakra produced its own extraordinary effects. Heart chakra, however, proved the most gentle and healing of the chakras so far. The practice of giving, receiving, forgiveness, love and gratitude was a soft and nourishing practice, far subtler than the fire of third chakra.

Thank you. Thank you for Sophie. For Reiki. Thank you for not giving up. I can only imagine yours was not an easy road to travel. Thank you for sharing this gift with me.

I was about to return my gaze to my binder, when several petals spontaneously released from one of the roses, dropping directly onto his photo. I jumped in my seat, startled.

"Did you see that?" Everyone spoke at once.

I admitted my lapse in focus from the course material, telling the group I had been giving thanks to its founder. The four of us were abuzz with awe; Sophie sat smiling, seemingly aware of the unseen guest in the room.

"It doesn't surprise me," she said.

The day floated by, filled with tea, sandwich wraps and the dark chocolate I contributed — my signature gift which, I admit, was really ever more for me than anyone else. I returned home briefly at lunch to prepare a gluten-free, dairy-free meal for the kids, an easier task for me than my mother-in-law since I had more practice. It was nice to see the kids in the midst of my dreamy day of energy studies. I kissed them goodbye and drifted back down the path to Sophie's.

Near the end of the afternoon, Sophie took us one by one into her treatment room. The treatment table removed, a single chair sat in the centre of the room. I smelled the distinct aroma of burning sage, a departure from her usual exotic essential oils. The sage indicated serious business afoot.

"Sit in the chair, please." Sophie smudged me with the sage, waving the smoke over my body, then continued with my Reiki attunement. "In order to allow healing energy to flow through your hands, we must open the palm chakras."

The entire process took only a few minutes.

"Golden hands," she said, holding both my hands in hers, palms facing up, as if she could see something I could not. I wafted out of the room with the aromatic plant smoke, and returned to my seat in the living room. The next student entered the treatment room.

I melted into the couch, thinking how a year earlier I knew nothing of chakras and how, in my year of yoga, they appeared at every turn, in every aspect of my life. They fascinated me, these colourful spinning wheels of energy. I couldn't see them, didn't understand how they worked, yet felt their connection to life, to health and healing, to rela-tionships, and emotions.

Even in my personal training work with clients, I had begun to see each person's issues as they moved in the studio. My mind no longer connected the movement to the muscle group or joint; instead it drew connections between restrictions in the body, the energy centres, and the issues involved with that chakra. Tight hips became less about hip flexors and glutes and more about issues of sexuality, play, creativity and emotional flow. I saw a weak core as issues of commitment, desire, fear and low inner fire. Tightness between the shoulder blades begged for self-love, nurturing and care.

I saw the interrelatedness of the mental, emotional, physical, and spiritual aspects of myself and others. Every thought rippled through us in some way. Every choice or emotion created some effect. If left unchecked, restriction began to form, blocking the energy like a dam. Leaks ensued, torrents raged and potential tsunamis lurked.

The door to the den opened and Sophie returned to the living room, along with the last of the students to receive an attunement. We hugged our good-byes in peace. I grabbed one last square of dark chocolate from the coffee table and popped it in my mouth to melt slowly on the walk home.

My senses were open, my mind clear, my heart full. Would this feeling remain or would it be like attending a motivational workshop; where, after a few days, the high wears off? My regular practice of yoga, meditation and affirmations had kept me on the path through my chakra inquiries. Sophie had suggested an additional daily practice of self-Reiki, to become familiar with the process and heighten my sense of energy. I committed to adding Reiki to my practice.

While Steve drove his mom home, I got the kids ready for bed. Michael started pushing boundaries. He was unwilling to cooperate with bath, pyjamas or teeth-brushing. The more I encouraged his cooperation, the harder he pushed against me. Finally, his defiance triggered my programmed response and I walked into his room to yell at him to get into bed. I opened my mouth to raise my voice, which usually elicited the desired response from him. I awaited the flush of heat to my face that precedes and fuels the yell. It never arose. I was unable to move to anger at that moment; it didn't exist in me. My mouth was open but nothing came out.

I picked Michael up and tucked him under his blankets, kissed him on the head and said goodnight. I didn't know how long my calm would last, if it was a result of my blissful day, the attunement, or both. Perhaps peace would come and go but the fact that I experienced that feeling of peace amidst drama, anticipating a conditioned reaction, showed me first-hand how powerful the practices were that I was discovering. I could no longer presume anything; the rules of the game had changed. I was changing along with them.

37

A PROFESSIONAL OPINION

Seven months had passed since the MRI and I finally received my appointment to officially review the results at the back clinic. I was grateful Aunt Joyce had shared her professional opinion with me months earlier, catapulting me into my year of exploration and discovery. If I had waited the seven months for the specialist, I would not have known Joyce's advice about moving from weights to yoga. When things aren't turning out the way you expect, sometimes you simply need to surrender and assume there is something bigger and better at play.

I sat in the waiting room in my fourth chakra attire — rose pink yoga top and electric pink track jacket — I was definitely the brightest one in the room. A choker necklace of pink pukka shells completed my ensemble. I sensed the mood of those waiting: the way they sat, slumped in their seats, head down or chin sunk into their hand. Dour expressions on their faces spoke to their pain or worry. Some sat patiently reading the newspaper, less engaged in the waiting process and its affinity for exponentially increasing anxiety. I smiled whenever someone caught my gaze, and continued people-watching, wondering what challenges each of them faced. Drunk on heart chakra, I wished them well, sending etheric lotuses through the air.

"Stephanie."

I followed the man holding my file into a room with a treatment bed on one side, a chair next to it and a computer desk opposite.

"My job is to assess your range of motion and level of pain," he said. "I'll make recommendations to the doctor, who will see you once we're done."

I lifted my arms and legs in sequences as he instructed. Then I repeated the movements while he applied resistance. Trying to raise my leg behind me in the air while he pressed down on my foot proved to be the most difficult of all the exercises. I sailed through the toe-touching forward bends and lateral reaches. I sat on the bed as he jotted notes in my file and loaded my MRI results onto the computer. He left the room, and returned shortly with an older gentleman, the specialist. We shook hands and the doctor pulled the chair up to the computer to review the MRI.

"I just saw a patient before you with a similar injury," he said. "That fellow shuffles around in pain, unable to work." The doctor scrolled images across the screen. "My team reviews results each week and makes recommendations as to which patients need to see the surgeon for further assessment." More scrolling. "If I were to make my recommendation based on the MRI alone, I would send you to the surgeon. However, seeing you in person, mobile, flexible, with a reasonably low level of pain, I question whether to refer you at all. I'll discuss it with the surgeon and, if necessary, we'll call you to set up an appointment to assess you for surgery."

My back felt good, my daily practices helped. Surgery

seemed unnecessary, yet the MRI images appeared serious. Grateful for the miracle of modern medicine, I didn't want to rule out a procedure that could be beneficial and necessary; however, my default position on medical procedures was that they be considered only as a last resort. I liked to exhaust natural remedies first. *I do not want to have to make the decision on whether or not to have surgery. Please let someone wise make this decision for me.*

The specialist leaned toward me in his chair, his elbows resting on his knees. "Once in a while a case exists where a patient recesses the bulge and makes a complete recovery," he said. "I believe you could be one of those cases."

He didn't have to share that with me. I thanked him. He planted a seed, rather, he watered a seed that I had planted. Someone who specialized in my particular health issue believed I could heal. It inspired and motivated me to continue my work.

He also spoke of elderly deceased patients whose autopsies revealed severe spinal injuries; yet, they'd experienced little discomfort in daily life. Their unknown physical states held no power over their ability to function. Perhaps ignorance *is* bliss. Maybe the mind holds more power over our pain than we realize.

"Stephanie, how is it that you are so mobile?"

"Daily yoga," I answered. I assumed the doctor would accept that answer over a lengthy story of how I was part of a group that explored our chakras through a variety of practices: physical, mental and spiritual. I imagined how that conversation would go:

"So, what's your secret?"

"Oh, you know, ... sitting in a salted circle on the lawn with Buddha and lighting shit on fire."

38

THROWING STONES

Steve and I cleaned up the dinner dishes and shared about the day. I vented my concerns of the week, overwhelmed by obligations: clients, kids, school, parent council meetings. I may have scraped a serving of real estate off my full plate, but I'd replaced it with a heaping helping of volunteer positions.

Holding the tea towel in hand, standing next to the kitchen island, Steve offered an observation. "It's like you are treading water and people keep coming to you, handing you rocks and asking you to hold them, promising to come back; but they never come back and there you are: treading water, holding their rocks."

I laughed, but he was right. Not only had I been attending to all my own tasks, I had taken on the tasks of others, barely able to keep my head above water. Steve and I connected that night, in a way we hadn't in a long time, and he helped me to see myself. His channeling of Confucius and accurate portrayal of me, resonated. It spurred me to begin my own forty-day inquiry while still in the inquiry of heart chakra. An inquiry within an inquiry — how Shake-spearean.

I put Steve's observation to the test; I lightened my load, yoga-style. Forty days of saying "No." Any email request from the school, a friend, or even a client, I responded to with "No." My sense of responsibility and commitment screamed in protest. It was hard on my head, but easier than I thought it would be because there were no other options. I knew the answer would have to be "No." Like the pendulum, I gave any decisions or contemplation over to one simple action: "No." I even ditched previous commitments which left me feeling guilty. I chose the inquiry and I committed to its process above all else. And magic happened.

My metaphoric pendulum of commitments had swung too far in one direction. As I swung it all the way to the other during the inquiry, it finally came to rest at centre. I began to notice my gut reaction when a request came. Knowing the answer already, no internal debate occurred. When I felt relieved at the no, my body relaxed, like I'd dodged a bullet. When I felt disappointed to say no, it was usually accompanied by a groan, sigh, or "Shit, I would have liked that." My body's response helped me tune in to my heart and my passions, not my sense of duty or appearance.

By the end of the inquiry and the forty days, I dropped all sorts of rocks and waded out of the water. I had devel-oped a good sense of when I was simply holding out my hand to accept another rock. I felt guilt-free in my subse-quent nay-saying as I respected and appreciated my body's messages and rhythms. Then a funny thing happened. People stopped asking me to hold their rocks.

39

FINDING MY MALA

I parked my car in a parking lot on the west side of the city, near the highway. Anna pulled into a spot next to me and I hopped into the backseat of her car, next to Karen. Anna's mom, in town for a visit, sat in the passenger seat.

We arrived at the Saddledome to find a long lineup. We parked and joined the line. The sun warmed me once the line crept out of the shade into its path. We spotted Alora and looked around for anyone else we knew. A variety of people had gathered, some in colourful garb, with ornate bags slung over their shoulders or tucked under arms, some were in business attire, and many wore jeans.

Nearly eighteen thousand people lined up to listen to His Holiness, the Fourteenth Dalai Lama, speak in Calgary's largest arena. Much anticipation had built around his visit; there was a sense that something profound was about to change in our city and the Dalai Lama held the key. It was as if he blessed our city, touched our hearts and graced our land; he left the door open for more love, compassion and spirituality to emerge, and more enlightened teachers to follow.

We had planned to arrive early as we heard security for the His Holiness was tight. Evidently, all other attendees heard the same. Truthfully, I was more interested in arriving ahead of time so I could shop the Dalai Lama's gift shop. *Prayer beads for everyone for Christmas!*

Inside the concourse, I settled on three charms; *Ganesha*, *hamsa* and a silver *Om* symbol with a single turquoise stone. I bought a hanging prayer banner for the studio, entitled *Never Give Up*. And I picked out one simple strand of mala beads. I was poised to meet one of my favourite people on the planet. Someone who's smile, strength, wisdom, compassion, and humour inspired, assured and encouraged me to move forward through life even when life on the planet didn't always make sense.

When His Holiness first came on to the stage, he acknowledged that people seek him for a variety of reasons. He stressed that he was not a healer I couldn't help but be honest about feeling judgmental of those who flocked to see His Holiness to be healed, but I was no different.

We all searched for something, some way to make sense of our lives, of the world. A secret or method of avoiding or rising above the struggle. The majority of us in attendance were looking for some way to heal ourselves: physically, mentally and spiritually; someone to connect us; to reconnect us to each other and some common goal to work toward; someone with the answers to our questions.

I had told Steve when we first met that there were a couple prominent people of our time that I wanted to see. Luciano Pavarotti was one and the Dalai Lama was the other. Seven years earlier, Steve and I had sat, rows away from Pavarotti, my eyes closed and tears streaming down my cheeks as *Nessun Dorma* transformed the room and my spirit. Sitting in the presence of the Dalai Lama filled me in the same way the great tenor's voice had; whether he answered my questions or not didn't matter.

I sent him gratitude as I watched and listened. Honestly, at the beginning of his address, I nodded off twice, partly because I was exhausted and partly due to his accent. Eventually my ears attuned to his speech and, by watching him closely, I could follow his words better, especially if I watched on the jumbotron. *Who booked the great man into the sports arena?* It took effort to enjoy His Holiness in the same venue where we cheered on "Our Calgary Flaaaaaaaaames." Of course, no other venue could have supported such a crowd.

Seeing him on the big screen did make his words easier to follow. When the Dalai Lama spoke, every word exuded consciousness. I was reminded that it was all about compassion, love, and looking deep within ourselves for the answers; it was about honouring ourselves and our children. One of the most interesting things for me was: I learned about his meditation practice.

The Dalai Lama said he meditated for approximately five to six hours per day. *Per day!* I was happy to commit to twenty minutes in the morning and again in the evening. I wondered if it was possibly a *get what you pay for* scenario. If you put in twenty minutes, you get twenty minutes'-worth. If you put in five hours, you get five hours'-worth. Five hours wasn't an option for me. I needed to balance daily life with children, family, play and work.

Toward the end of the evening, His Holiness asked that the lights in the arena be turned up so he could see to whom he spoke and we could see one another. The lights came up and I saw thousands of people gathered in community, all wearing the white prayer scarves received when we entered the arena. The Dalai Lama asked us to hold the ends of the scarves worn by the people on either side of us.

I took the ends of Karen's and Anna's and they took mine. In that moment, eighteen thousand people connected with each other and His Holiness — a spiritual community in a hockey arena — each a bead in a human mala.

40

A WHOLE LOTTA' LOVE

Most days began with lotus offerings for Steve, the kids and myself, in gratitude. If anyone else came to mind during the sun salutations, I offered them a lotus as well. Some mornings, I needed to cap the line-up. Once I opened the gates, people flooded my mind for a blessing. Who couldn't use more gratitude?

Each time I completed the practice, warmth and happiness filled my heart and home. I let go of days when early morning practice was side-tracked by kids up at night or up too early. I was easy on myself if practice didn't happen, moving forward with my day gently and not dragging the missed practice along with it.

I completed my practice with thirty minutes of self-Reiki. Lying on the floor, I hovered my hands over my body, scanning and noticing any sensations in my hands — warmth or tingling — as I sent myself love. Most times, I woke to find my hands collapsed somewhere on my body; I could tell how far I'd gotten before nodding off, by their location. I figured it all worked out and I benefited from both the daily practice and the nap.

This particular day was different. I opened the window of the living room, craving fresh air. I lay down on my back on the carpet, hands over face: warmth. Hands over throat: energy moving.

But, then there's a glass. A crystal glass with a sunflower etched on the side. It's half-full of iced tea, still bubbling from the soft farm water. The nostalgic fragrance of lilacs fills my nose. They stand, freshly cut, in a round crystal bowl etched with the same sunflower. The lilacs mingle with pink peonies. A lone ant searches the petals frantically for kin. The sun streams in through the large windows that boast a view of fields and barns, and the vast stretch of white fences, painted by my cousins and me one summer. We painted the fence boards, the grass, ourselves, each other, and most likely a horse or two in the process.

The midday newscaster informs of the local events on the small kitchen television while Nan sits at the table with the day's paper. She works the crossword puzzle with a slightly shaky but elegant hand, and produces equally elegant letters in cursive.

"What's new in your young life?" she asks, and I feel as if everything is right with the world.

I woke to find one hand across my chest and the other on the floor, the details still fresh in my mind. More so, my heart.

The farm kitchen was long gone, as were days of crosswords with Nan. But the overwhelming feelings of comfort, happiness, contentment, and love remained, though often hidden. They were not found in salt crystal lamps or essential oils. Those feelings were not found in the *what*, but the *who*.

My heart was opening. My most cherished memories were also my saddest losses: life on the farm, a childhood of playing in nature, endless summer days and iced tea with Nan. I had sealed the warmth of the memories in with the pain of the loss. Love and grief are familiar dance partners.

Days in heart chakra ended with eleven minutes of alternate-nostril breathing followed by silent chanting of *aham prema* The practice of *Metta Bhavana,* offering blessings and well wishes to someone I loved — living or dead — a casual acquaintance, someone with whom I struggled, and myself, completed the set.

"Nan, may you be happy. May you be healthy. May you be safe. May you be free from inner and outer suffering. May you live with ease and joy." My grief was gently held somewhere between *metta* for Nan and *metta* for Stephanie.

I enjoyed thinking back over my day to find someone I encountered to send an anonymous blessing. At first, my blessings for a difficult person were equally difficult. More smiling heart was required. As my practice continued, I found it less and less challenging to bestow good wishes upon someone with whom I struggled. In that, my heart expanded further. It was I who healed through the practice.

Soaking in the bath, candle lit, lavender-scented salts dissolving around me, I sank into the water up to my chin, closed my eyes and thought of all those I needed to forgive.

"I forgive you," I whispered in the water after each name — no details, no conditions, no memories, no story — simple and complete forgiveness.

"For a person who cherishes compassion and love, the practice of tolerance is essential, and for that, an enemy is indispensable. So we should be grateful to our enemies, for it is they who can best help us develop a tranquil mind." ~His Holiness, the Dalai Lama

PART VI

THROAT CHAKRA

COMMUNICATE

Before you can speak,
you need to learn to listen.

41

VISHUDDHA... GUZUNTIGHT

I inhaled the earthy aroma of fallen leaves, damp with early morning dew. The cool air stung my throat, already raw with infection — part of the Kundalini journey, I guessed, as we gathered for fifth chakra, throat chakra. A small tabby cat crossed the lane in front of the lodge and sat under a tractor, rubbing its scent on the heavily-treaded tire. I crouched down and extended my hand to lure the cat.

She slowly swaggered toward me in typical feline fashion. I scratched under her chin as Nurse Louise and Britt approached the porch and we exchanged warm greetings, happy to see one another. No longer strangers, we were friends — more than friends; we'd become a community.

I gathered my yoga bag and we entered the lodge; we removed our shoes and jackets in the entrance and mindfully placed them in the wooden coat cubby. Warm spices wafted around the corner as I entered the large kitchen. Alora stood at the double sink, preparing tea for the morning's sharing. The ritual of tea soothed my senses; the warmth of the mug cupped in both hands, the aroma of citrus and cinnamon, the hot liquid on my lips. Like a child with a blanket, I found great comfort in a cup of tea.

Only four of us gathered for fifth chakra. Others fell too ill or had other commitments. My throat burned, but I refused to miss a gathering. I soothed my suffering with tea. The cabin seemed empty without the full group, yet intimate. I slipped into the serenity of the soft morning like a hot bath.

We began our practice with focus on our voice and how we used it to communicate with ourselves and others. My voice sounded rough and scratched my throat as it passed through.

We began our practice with focus on communication: how we used our voice to talk to ourselves and others. We started by evaluating our excuses. We used Wayne Dyer's new book, *Excuses Begone!*, to identify and examine our common excuses. We then spoke aloud the affirmations related to them.

As I rifled through the many choices, I realized I was in a good place. Not a lot of excuses held me back from achieving what I wanted in life. I did, however, take a long pause on the *family* card of excuses.

Sitting at fifth chakra, a new winter looming, I pondered family as my excuse for not moving forward to discover my life's purpose. I had left real estate to focus on family. I wrestled and wrangled my ego and self-importance to find harmony in my home. Was I also using family as an excuse to not realize my highest potential?

I spent a couple seconds on the money excuse card. Let's face it, who couldn't accomplish great things with a lot of money? As I learned in third chakra, fear almost always rested at the root of an issue, and fear of lack, lack of money, rested at the root of issues for me. Not as deeply rooted as family or identity or authenticity, but still rooted.

The family fear looked something like this: afraid to get to the end of my life not having achieved what I came here to do because I was wrapped up in family. Or, getting to the end of my life, having achieved all the other stuff that seemed important, only to realize family was what I came here to experience. And why did it have to be one or the other? Social conditioning provided the fertilizer for the family versus work debate. The mind's propensity for duality provided the struggle.

I had money. Not as much as my ego wished, but we were fortunate enough to want for nothing of importance. Thanks, largely, to Steve's work ethic, all our needs were met. All our material needs — which had slowly become a source of agitation for me. The accumulation of *things* had become little more than clutter once I understood that the fortune I lacked was spiritual, not monetary. Too much stuff.

We shared our excuses and recorded them in our journals, along with the prescribed affirmations. Time to move our bodies. We headed to our mats to begin our fifth chakra yoga practice. Throat opening poses and lion's breath warmed us up.

"I speak for myself. I speak from my heart. I allow my skills and creativity to be expressed and voiced to the world," Alora gave the affirmations.

"Fifth chakra is your voice, communication, expression and personal truth," Alora said as she guided us into cobra pose. "Speak from the heart. Be silent long enough and often enough to allow authentic expression to surface ... then express yourself honestly and clearly."

Throat chakra addressed verbal diarrhea — too much chatter without purpose, intent or clarity. Our words could be used as medicine or weapons. Fifth chakra, *vishuddha*, Sanskrit for *purification*: our throat channel could either ease struggle in our life and that of others through words, or create further struggle.

Fifth chakra was the first of the chakras to focus primarily on the spiritual plane. Ether or *akasha*, meaning *space*, is the element of throat chakra. The colour associated with it is blue, as in clear blue sky. Creativity and self-expression reside in fifth chakra. In throat chakra, feelings and emotions take form in sound, words, writing and expression.

Channeling words, writing, music, song, and communicating with animals or across realms is possible in throat chakra. Communication through other levels of consciousness — dream yoga and lucid dreaming – are associated with fifth chakra.

Fish pose, cobra, shoulder stand and rabbit opened our throats and necks and occupied much of our morning and our asana focus. We lingered in savasana, then sat for a long period of silence. My swollen throat welcomed the reprieve.

We broke for lunch later than usual and enjoyed a modest potluck since our numbers were few. My contribution was neither vegetarian nor healthy: signature cupcakes from the most popular bakery in the city, to celebrate both my birthday and Anna's — four days apart and the week after our gathering. Since Anna didn't make it to the group, I saved a few cupcakes to drop off at her house on my way back to the city.

Britt brought an enormous homemade apple strudel, a sight to behold. A decadent dessert buffet indulged our throat chakra and our small group. We washed it down with spicy chai tea. We savoured lunch as we had savoured our practice: slowly and dreamily. After lunch, we opened our throat chakra to chant the mantra we would repeat over the next forty days: *Om Mani Padme Hum*.

We chanted the sacred mantra, cornerstone to Tibetan Buddhist practices, in unison with the voices emerging through the speakers of Alora's sound system. The music continued, turning to crystal bowls and Tibetan throat singing. We chanted *Om* along with the monks, deep, long, slow, low, *ooooommmmmmmmmmmmmm*. My lips vibrated, my cheekbones, earlobes, eyes, ribcage and scalp all resonated with the sound emanating from my throat and breath.

The chanting continued, morphing into the mantra *ham*, the seed sound for throat chakra. I filled my lungs with breath to feed the mantra's appetite. *Huuuuuuummmmmm-mmm*. After several minutes of chanting we used our open throat chakras to vibrate all our chakras — consciously climbing the ladder as we chanted the seed sound for each energy center.

Lam, vam, ram, yam, ham, aaaaauuuuuuummmmm, we chanted, my body numbing, every cell reverberating the monotonous vibrations of the synthesis of sound and breath. My head pulsed electric with the current of sound. After what seemed like hours of humming, chanting and vibrating, we fell into quiet, eyes closed. My body continued to vibrate, the residue of the long vishuddha practice. The silence accentuated my hyper-awareness to the frequency of my body and my surroundings. My spidey senses tingled. I felt crystal clear, no thoughts, no chatter, no noise. My body echoed *hum* in the silence.

"Open your eyes and bring movement into your body." Alora's voice sifted through the space. She led us outside to walk around Sacred Forest and spend time in nature.

After our walk, we each found a place to sit and write. I found myself at Gabriella's trampoline, near the main house. I lay across it, opening my journal to a fresh blank page. Tiny snowflakes danced onto the paper and I pulled my zipper to the top of my jacket, tucking my chin into my collar. I composed a poem while two of Gabriella's cats walked the perimeter of the trampoline in high-wire-artist style. I wrote my poem to Magpie, who perched on the fence, and who, I realized, had accompanied me through life.

The Tibetan tingshas rang in the distance. Alora called us back to the cabin. "Don't go into the sunroom. Wait here. No peeking. I have a surprise for you."

We slipped off our outer wear and silently sipped tea in the kitchen while Alora returned again and again to place a blindfold on each of us. She led us by the hand, one at a time, into the sunroom. I slid my foot across the hardwood floor before me. *Slow down, lady.* I waved one hand out in front to identify anything before I ran into it, the other hand held by Alora as she walked ahead.

"Watch the door frame as we enter the sunroom." She led me to my mat. "Lie down or sit in a comfortable position."

I wondered what she had cooked up for us, always a surprise with Alora. I felt the hardwood on my shoulder blades and across the back of my pelvis. I shifted on my mat in the muted blackness of the blindfold, listening to others take their places, then Alora settling in. The room fell still. I heard my breath and relaxed into the familiar savasana position, alert to what may come.

A high note sliced the air, gradually building in volume as the unmistakeable voice of a crystal bowl sang out. Another voice joined in: the low hum of a larger bowl. The vibrations entered my back body. Multiple bowls bounced sound waves off hardwood and walls. My bones reached for the pulsing wood. I sank into my mat and the floor and surrendered deeply to the sounds. Time ceased to exist while I travelled on the waves.

My year had shifted somewhere. After third chakra, after heart gathering, the journey changed for me. Every day I woke to a slightly altered reality, all within. My bed the same, my work the same, my breakfast the same, but my perception had changed. I felt less of the previous strain of physical existence

I slept deeply on my mat, although possibly not at all, ceasing to exist in thought and form for the duration of the sound bath. No memory, no drooling, no snoring. As the bowls' voices slowly faded, I drifted back into my body, as if I'd been away for years. Unable to move any part of me, I remained with my breath until it deepened enough to reanimate my body and allow me to open my eyes and shift into a seated position.

A petite woman dressed in white, with shoulder-length black hair sat, surrounded by soft pink crystal bowls of all sizes. Candles surrounded the bowls, illuminating them with soft light. All sat on a large white cloth with ornately embroidered edges. Alora formally introduced our crystal musician as Lily and asked her to share her story.

"I learned to work with the crystal bowls from a great teacher. He gave me the bowls and we played brilliantly, the bowls and I. Then the teacher came back one day and asked for the bowls. I lost them that day. Years later, they found their way back to me. It was a bittersweet reunion. I resisted playing them. They sat in storage. Just recently I found my voice again, and theirs, and I agreed to share them with everyone."

Our group humbly thanked Lily for sharing her gift and art, and then refreshed our tea for the final practice of the day: stringing our commitment bracelets. I slipped each round, blue, sodalite bead onto the string with intentions of communication, truth, finding my voice, creative expression, writing, silence and creating space for the new to enter my life. I filled each bead with intentions of *vishuddha*.

THE FOG RETURNS

Two weeks into throat chakra practice, my throat had nearly healed. But, I was blessed with a sinus infection and the barely tolerable pain at the base of my skull. The next level of kundalini energy had begun to emerge. With a long overdue trip for Steve and me planned, the sinus infection needed to remain low key, at least until after the excursion.

Although excited to get away with Steve, I still craved a spiritual escape in our trip. We planned to travel to San Francisco for a weekend with our neighbours, leaving Michael and Khali with my mom and dad. Meditating by the Bay would be poor social form, so I complied with dinner reservations and wine tastings. I did manage to locate a little crystal shop online that sold Reiki healing crystals to satisfy my itch for the mystical.

The breath-taking surroundings of the vineyards and California countryside spoke my language. Our day tour into wine country with our neighbours shone. However, I succumb to complaining on day three, when I found myself doing what I thought we *should* do in the famous city: shopping. What I really wanted to do was yoga.

At the same time, I was hyper-aware of awareness. *Am I supposed to find something meaningful in this store? Did we wander into this neighbourhood for a reason?* And because of the craziness in my brain, I dropped over two hundred and fifty dollars on Reiki stones and crystals in the crystal shop. Fifth chakra ran rampant, yet I never articulated to myself or others what I really wanted out of the trip.

I craved a yoga class. Even if that meant asking my husband to spend a couple hours finding something of his own to do. I enjoyed shopping, but I'd had enough of the pavement, people and street noise.

Steve and I jumped on the trolley on our final evening, free from our travelling companions, feet sore from a day's walking and shopping.

"Forget finding a local gem of a restaurant," I said. "I'm starving. Let's just grab the nearest food we can find."

"There's not much here," Steve searched the street through the trolley window. "Wait. There's a hotel. Wanna jump off?"

"Sure."

"It's only five o'clock."

"So, it'll be us, senior citizens, and people with young children dining." I laughed. Steve smiled.

We stepped into the hotel restaurant, happy to get off our feet. The waiter seated us at a quiet table — not a difficult feat, since the restaurant proved near-empty.

"I'll have water with lemon, please," I said.

"Same. No lemon though," added Steve.

More conversation was exchanged with the waiter than between my husband and me.

Finally, my fifth chakra cleared. "I feel like we kinda' wasted this day," I said.

"Yeah, me too."

"I would have loved to do a yoga class or two today. San Fran is the yoga mecca of the U.S."

"You *should've*. I'd have been fine with that. I could've spent a couple hours in the Apple store while you took a class."

"I wish we'd have had this conversation earlier. It's been so long since we've had time alone without the kids, I felt like we should spend it together."

"I know. Me too." Steve reached for my hand across the table.

"I'd have been good with you taking time to do your own thing, you know ... Apple Store or otherwise."

"Next time," Steve said. "Let's enjoy our dinner." And we did just that; we enjoyed our dinner, amidst the sparse tables of seniors and young families.

The next day, we realized we should have checked in at the airline earlier, online. We ended up with seat assignments in the last row on the plane, and not together. I stewed at the gate.

"Why don't you go ask for a first class bump?" Steve egged me on. "Like you used to."

I finally approached the gate agent for an upgrade. "Hi, I noticed I am in the last row on the aircraft and understand those seats don't recline."

"Yes, that row is situated next to the lavatory. There is limited movement of the seats."

"Are there any other available seats on the aircraft? I have a back injury and the inability to recline my seat is going to make for an excruciating flight." Okay, I milked the injury. "As well, my husband and I have been seated apart. I would really appreciate any other seats you have to offer."

Many years in sales had taught me that, when negotiating, there was a time to talk and a time to shut up. While the gate agent clicked away at her keyboard, it was time to shut up. I gave her the space to do what she needed to do.

"Hmmm. I have two seats remaining on the aircraft," she said and continued to click. I continued to hold my tongue. *Give her space.* She printed the tickets and handed them to me. "For you and your husband."

"I can't thank you enough." I smiled and took the tickets. I resisted glancing at them until I had reached Steve. I slipped him a sly smile.

"No way," he grabbed the tickets.

Last two seats on the plane. First class.

We flew home in style and celebrated the last leg of our trip together. And maybe messaged a selfie of us clinking champagne flutes from first class to our neighbours seated in economy. Communicating what I needed to the gate agent paid off. Propped on pillows, cozy under blankets, snacks and drinks in hand, Steve enjoyed a movie while I caught up on my reading of *A New Earth*. The plane cleared the runway and the Bay as the fog cleared from my marriage.

43

THE ENERGY OF AN ILLNESS

In the midst of the great influenza (H1N1) pandemic's vaccination program, I found fifth chakra. I had stopped watching the news and reading the paper during my year in yoga, as I preferred to guide the energy of my day through *my* choices of vibrations: music, mantra, yoga, the outdoors, baking and cooking, writing, reading, or musing about all things supernatural. I had unplugged from the media to plug into myself.

If I sat with the doom and gloom of the world, I became snagged on it and paralyzed to do anything about it. If I focused on my contribution to my family and community, and putting my best and strongest self forward, I overcame the paralysis. I didn't need to see the world through rose-coloured glasses; I needed inspiring stories of real people and communities working to create solutions.

As the H1N1 vaccine camps set up around town, it became better entertainment than *America's Got Talent*. Debates popped up about it on Facebook. Conversations were overheard in the supermarket, schools, office, every-where. A steady stream of information flowed home from school in Michael's backpack, and my inbox was flooded with forwarded emails on the subject.

"The lab confirmed it: H1N1." My friend was the first case that became personal for me. This strain of influenza proved real. What became interesting to me was, the more I watched, talked about and read about it, the worse I felt: fear, frustration, helplessness, the victim, paralyzed.

My yogic bliss gone, my body, heavy and lethargic, matched my mood. I debated each day over the vaccine; I was angry, frustrated and confused. I felt no need to vaccinate myself or my children, yet my mind filled with *what ifs* and worse case scenarios, and a need to continually research and fact find.

The news portrayed two camps — the vaccinators and the non-vaccinators — driving the *us-against-them* mentality where nobody wins. I wouldn't touch the debate on vaccination. People became passionate about their stance and things got heated. I simply wanted to make the best decision for myself and my family. Everything about the situation, the state of the community, felt strained, damp, dark and frightened.

Emails even came from our yoga community, however, they promoted *nasya*, nutrition, rest, supplementation, and herbal support — a different take, yet still proving the impact and reach of the pending pandemic. One online article addressed the benefits of pranayama, yoga and Ayurveda in preventing and treating flu and colds. As I read the article and explored the kriya, I started practicing the breathing.

My energy shifted as if I'd shed a heavy coat or blanket. With every breath, more weight lifted and I began to feel and see more clearly. I had slowly allowed myself to get sucked back into a low vibration driven by negativity. I returned to breath, to affirmation, to lightness of being, to a state that allowed me to connect with myself and the answers right for me at the time.

I sat quietly after the breath work, and pondered the issue. *Would changing the paths of my thoughts keep me from getting sick? Not sure.* Didn't really care just then. What I cared about was the mind driving, fear-based thought, and becoming a victim to each negative detail it grabbed ahold of.

I turned off the news, closed my laptop lid, and reaffirmed my practice. My mind clear, ease returned to my body, thoughts and breath. I was accused of sticking my head in the sand. It was *my* head and my conscious choice where to stick it, my truth. My thoughts affected my energy, tying my stomach in knots with worry and fear, draining my energy, and leaving me deflated — crushed beneath a wave of collective fear.

The kriya, the breathing, the momentary detachment from the situation, eased my body and mind and, from that place, I could make the best choice. I needed to feel what I experienced and acknowledge what I felt. I needed to choose what to do with my feelings and how to proceed. My main concern was for my kids' health and well-being. I needed to model for them and make the best choices I knew.

The phrase *energy flows where attention goes* played in my head. I saw how the media frenzy, the intense energy of the community, the city, the province, the country, the world even, affected my energy. I also saw how, when I made a choice to remove myself and go within, I shed the effects and returned to a more balanced state. I focused on the best course of action for my family.

44

MAMA'S BOY

A clever and independent kid, I often assigned Michael a lot of responsibility, helping me with Khali, the groceries and tasks around the house, and I tended to forgot how young he was. Always eager to take on a new challenge, Michael had complied with most requests. Initially, it was fun to teach him to help out, but as I became tired, I found I demanded more of Michael, and felt less enthusiastic about making it fun. Michael had vied for attention from me, uninterrupted by the tiny interloper he knew as his baby sister; I struggled to find time for myself, let alone my husband, each child individually, and the family as a whole.

The year's inquiries proved nourishing for me and the family, and I felt ease and peace restored in myself and my home. Still, the habitual impatience lingered with Michael and I wished to communicate better with him. During my new moon meditation two weeks earlier, I had focused my intention on family harmony.

I woke this morning to discover something had shifted over the past weeks. I lay in bed feeling different about my relationship with Michael. Not sure exactly how, I reviewed how we had related to one another over the past couple weeks. We had experienced a gradual shift: me more patient, and him more responsive.

When I considered my relationship with my husband, and how my children had blossomed, I realized that the year focused on *family* through yoga, had transformed me. Content with my relationship with Michael, knowing it wasn't an all-the-time event and we would still have our moments of frustration, I accepted that those moments contained the seeds to grow together. I held awareness around how we could improve, allow, accept and forgive each other as we supported, nurtured, celebrated and loved one another. There was harmony in my home.

Because of the work on myself, because of my own happiness, I approached Michael and everyone from a different place, and they, in turn, responded. I stopped expecting happiness to come from others. I stopped demanding everyone else did as I said in order for me to be content. Most importantly, I began to see my reactivity to others, and how easily peace could be lost by my reaction to someone else's actions.

Not always easy, I focused on my response to my family members, encouraging them to communicate their needs, wants and feelings while plumbing the depths of mine and untying my reaction from theirs. A difficult practice, not getting caught up in someone else's drama, yet holding compassion and empathy for them. I felt the practice would yield gold if I mastered it.

Everyone was simply seeking their happiness in any given moment, as I sought my own. It was hard to disparage someone else their process. Depending upon how much noise filled my brain, I either happily allowed Michael his freedom to express and yell and let off steam or sing at the top of his lungs, or I yelled back at him, "Go to your room! No singing at the table! Indoor voice!" Honestly, if a child can't sing over a good meal with family, then we've lost something we need to recover. When my mind was calm, my tongue was calm. When my mind was loud, so was my voice.

Frustration melted away and no longer found the kids as targets. If the source of my frustration revealed Steve, I asked myself further questions: *Is it him or something I want from him?* Breathing centred me and allowed me to assess if my agitation was real and required a conversation between us, or if I simply needed to let it go.

Communication within my home and family changed because I changed the way I communicated. It started and ended with me. Ultimately no one else derailed me unless I allowed it — a difficult concept in a family unit with everyone sharing space nearly every moment of the day, but I felt it to be true.

If I could master *me*, my communication, and reactions, calm could reside in every moment, regardless of the situation. I also knew, as the centre of the home, Mom held the potential for the energy of the home. If Mom was happy, everyone was happy, or at least if Mom was calm and content, she didn't blow up the house.

45

BREATHING THROUGH IT

W e all came down with H1N1, except Steve. Michael requested if I could "do that thing Sophie taught you." He asked for Reiki, typically falling asleep during the short treatment.

"Mom, can you do that thing *every* night? I like how it feels. It helps me sleep."

"Of course I can. What exactly *do* you feel when I do that thing Sophie taught me?"

"I feel a beam of heat," he said.

His choice of words surprised me as Reiki is often described precisely that way by adults receiving treatment. I enjoyed working with Michael and him communicating his experience to me. He and I worked together to nurture each other.

I continued to play with crystals, symbols, healing vibrations and to connect to nature, with an underlying understanding that all I felt from those sources also existed within. Connecting with them amplified my innate ability to heal, as did connecting with Michael in Reiki, or with my community in yoga, or with Earth in meditation. I connected deeper when I chose not to seek.

The flu continued to be an unwanted guest in our house The kids, at the end of a mild case, enjoyed a couple days off school —watching movies and receiving evening Reiki sessions with me. Steve missed out entirely, which seemed to be the case with the men in many families we knew. I got the worst of it, but was surprised at how well I handled it.

I breathed and surrendered, rested and nurtured myself through every aching muscle, throbbing headache and even embraced the retching over the porcelain throne as a purification process. When my body ached, I relied on my breath to soothe it and when the waves of nausea crested, I drew deeply upon breath to move though the discomfort. *So hum*, I repeated in my head. I lay on the couch, cuddled in a blanket with a cup of tea, my fuzzy thoughts drifted to my first encounter with breathing through pain.

Ten years earlier I had flipped my mountain bike and flew head over heels over the handle bars, landing on the pavement. I remembered hearing the sound of my head strike the pavement, no helmet to cushion the blow. When I came to, a small crowd encircled me and a woman crouched over me. She placed her finger on my chest.

"Focus on breathing in and out," she had coached. "Concentrate on moving my finger up with the inhale and down with the exhale."

My head and neck felt hot and I immediately thought I must be bleeding out on the pavement. *Why else would my head be hot?* Aware of the multitude of signals and sensations running through my body, I didn't panic or try to get up. I listened to the woman's soothing voice. She said she was a nurse. I continued to breathe, hypnotically moving her finger up and down until the ambulance arrived.

I remember feeling every bump, every strip and patch of tar on the road, as pain shot through my body, but I remembered to breathe the breath she taught me. *They need to fix this damn stretch of highway.* A call came over the radio in the cab of the ambulance, a car accident farther up the highway toward Lake Louise. *How awful, someone might really be hurt.*

"If you need to attend to that," I'd told the paramedics. "I'll be alright."

They laughed at me. "Sure, we'll just leave you on the side of the highway and be back later to pick you up."

I remember countless x-rays on my head and having to heave myself on and off the exam table in excruciating pain, as the attendant was too tiny to support my weight. *Lovely girl. Maybe hire a bigger porter.*

I remembered many things from that day, none as clearly as the woman who placed her finger on my chest and taught me to breathe. Lucky to be alive, I had chosen that day to battle egos with my ex-husband who refused to wear a helmet. I had always worn mine — except for that day. I sure showed him.

Days later, once the vomiting subsided, I took cookies to the paramedics to say thank you. It was their job, but the smiles on their faces suggested that most days it was a thankless one. The person I wished to thank was the nurse who helped me breathe and reassured me with her presence.

～

AFTER I RECOVERED FROM H1N1, Anna and I laughed about our misery over the phone.

"Oh my God, Anna. I was hurling hard. And in between

I was like, *inhale I am, exhale clearing.* I think I'm good and purified!"

"Same," she replied. "Breathing got me through it."

The most important understanding I believe I had at that point in my year, was that there was no need to add or gain anything to move toward fulfillment. What I needed was to drop things, remove the interference in the channels, between the energy centres. Like radio waves, signals were best received if I first eliminated sources of interference. My signal was clearest when mind chatter, mouth chatter, and habitual behaviours were cleaned out.

Once a clear channel of communication, I needed to decide which frequency I wanted to connect to at any given moment. Sometimes I could do that simply with awareness. Other times, difficult times, I relied on my practices to face the muck and elevate me to preferred vibration. When I couldn't get myself into a full practice, I relied on my breath. It was always available.

46

DIGITAL DISTRESS

Opening my laptop was like opening the lid of Pandora's box: online shopping, email, Facebook. I preferred the organic feel of pen on paper, but unless I planned to publish my first work in handwritten ink I needed to eventually bring the laptop into the equation. The kids napped, the pot roast simmered in the oven, the incense smouldered on the mantle and I sat with a cup of tea, attempting to remember all that had happened over the previous sixty days.

I found little restraint with social media, succumbing to the temptation to read, scroll and comment far too often. I enjoyed many of the posts and pages about yoga, meditation, and various global conservation efforts, sharing them at will. Still, too much of my energy was wrapped up in digital "conversation".

A Facebook *friend* launched at me online one day, attacking my support of freedom of speech during the infamous Wikileaks. Hot under the collar, I readied retaliation. *How dare he attack my point of view. I didn't post on his shit.*

He'd never commented on my posts before. Why now? Why this one? Why so vehemently?

"Don't reply," Steve warned.

I deleted the reply I had so quickly banged out on my keyboard. I got up and walked away from my laptop. I continued to stew, poked by outrage. I rushed back to my laptop, clicking away again.

"Don't do it. Just leave it alone," insisted Steve. "Don't waste your energy on a response."

Of course he was right. But something in *me* wanted to be right too.

I left it. Left his comment to stand alone on my page for everyone to witness and for me to let be. Clearly his attack had little to do with me. His lengthy response cited a long list of fear-based remarks. Fuelling that fire would only make it grow hotter. I took many deep breaths to keep myself from crafting a stinging reply.

I began to understand conscious communication from a place of clarity and courage. Courage to speak out when needed, to keep silent when silence is warranted, courage to let go when fighting isn't the answer, and courage to hold compassion for someone who strikes out against me. I was not the true target of his attack, and understanding that, assisted my move toward compassion. A slow move, an inconsistent move, but a move nonetheless.

47

PSYCHE!

E mails flew the day before the retreat. So did the snow. Concerns over transportation, road closures and safety arose, as well as time conflicts as we neared Christmas. Several mates had fallen out of the boat, or rather, had disembarked at various ports along the way: Suzie got off at the port of career change; Fred departed at physical injury island, requiring time to heal his broken leg. We continued to include them in the group correspondence. Yvonne discovered the exotic port of new love and we wished her well. With so many missing, Alora combined the Saturday group and the Sunday group into one.

She settled on a start time of ten in the morning. Although our local roads remained largely impassible, I trusted my route would open up by morning and allow me to join the others. Lisa and I expressed our need to leave the retreat early. Alora conceded the evening's plan for an early dismissal so Lisa could pick up her kids and we could all get home before dark.

I woke to cleared roads, and patiently drove to the lodge.

I arrived at Sacred Forest to discover disappointing news. "I am guided to stay in fifth chakra longer," Alora said.

What? I had looked forward to sixth chakra, practically coveting the opportunity to explore all things psychic and unseen. Of course, I accepted Alora's decision. I had not yet fulfilled my writing goals for fifth chakra. The delay gifted me with an extension.

Still, I was disappointed. *I drove all the way out here for nothing. I could have stayed home, cozy in the snow globe that was my living room.*

We gathered in the cabin's living room with tea. A larger group, we filled the couches and chairs then spilled out onto floor cushions, leaning against those sitting on the furniture for comfort and support. I sat on the floor, resting against Anna's legs. Alora cued up a movie: *Enlighten Me.* The film about one man's journey into yoga suited our group.

It left me with the insight that even though our group shared similar events and often outcomes from our inquiries, every person walked his or her own path and experienced the same events differently. Sometimes we expected too much from an event or experience and other times we were not ready or open to receive more than what we got. We chose bite-sized chunks and either swallowed or spit them out. Radical change proved difficult for most people and small steps made change seem easier. Not everyone has that luxury. Some are forced to take great leaps due to sudden life change or emergency.

Alora gathered everyone in the sunroom after the movie. "We're going to experience a rant," she said. She stood in the middle of the standing circle. "One person will come into the centre while everyone else holds sacred space for them to express whatever wants to come out ... however it chooses to emerge."

No one moved. No one volunteered to go first. We stood, stunned. Then one brave soul jumped into the ring and it was game on. Ranting started slowly, softly and politely for some, erupting into great torrents of energy and emotions that had been suppressed. Others plunged directly into their turbulent waters, coming up briefly for air as they verbalized every detail of their frustration and pain.

My time came. *Great.* I was still grumpy about not moving onto sixth chakra. *Now I'm offered a soap box to get up on and air my crap? Perfect.* A build up of stuff began to pour forth from my lips. Maybe if I ranted once a month, Steve and the kids would no longer get hit with the residue of built-up emotions that dribbled at the least opportune time.

"Well, I'm not real happy about not moving forward in our year and the next chakra. I'm pretty pissed about people who refuse to open to sustainability and alternative ways of thinking and living. I'm somewhere between angry at my neighbour for attacking me online, and disappointed with myself for not letting him have it." My face heated as I moved around inside the circle, talking, in large part, with my hands. "But I know that would go nowhere. Nothing would be settled. No one would win. But it doesn't help my anger. What the fuck do I do with that? I feel compassion. But I also feel anger. I know I made the right choice, but I'm still left with the unresolved crap ... " I thought I'd dealt with that. Apparently not. Stuff flowed out after that. The rant faucet was wide open.

The heat remained in my face as the last person, Jill, entered and silently stood in the circle. She wept openly without a word. The circle stood firm, intent on securing a safe space for our wounded member to express and release her pain and sadness. I moved between fighting my own tears of empathy, and letting them flow for her, and me, and for us all.

Her sobbing filled the room. Every person in that circle felt for Jill. We held. Silent. Strong. Supportive. Her crying broke me open. It reached a place in me: a well of belonging, of humanity and collective suffering. It pulled the witness from me. I wore anger while Jill wore grief.

Expression exploded from our group: the freedom to speak our truths; to let go and let emotions and words fly; to reveal ourselves and our wounds, some wide open and raw; fortitude to stand guard for the other, respecting her space and her process while supporting her healing; wisdom to be silent, and to honour the silence of another. All of us were cleansed by the shower of tears; we completed the exercise, embracing Jill one by one before heading to the kitchen to replenish our tea. Deep breath.

Alora managed to find a last-minute replacement facilitator for a final afternoon exercise since our scheduled presenter had cancelled due to weather. A woman sat in one of the high-back chairs in the living room to share communications from nonphysical beings, namely angels and ancestors. The experience hinted at the sixth chakra essence I had hoped to explore that day.

The fire lit, tea in hand, we surrounded her as she asked us to invite any energies that wished to join us, in the form of those passed on or guardians in angelic form. I was more apt to believe in aliens than angels. Reiki had introduced me to angels and I continued to explore their presence.

Through the course of my many Reiki sessions and training, I had seen light of different colours and knew it as energy. I associated the energies with their angelic counterparts based on the colour of the light, but had yet to have one of the lights say, "Hello, my name is Raphael, how's it going?" I remained open and available for further communication.

The woman relayed messages to Gabriella from her dearly departed grandmother. And she answered questions from the group. I wrote down something she said, a Zen quote: *Before enlightenment, chop wood, carry water. After enlightenment, chop wood, carry water.* I assumed that as I became more aware and awake, life would become effortless. As the phrase sank in, I realized the effortlessness came from knowing the mind — no struggle, no strain — yet life's day-to-day tasks remained. I didn't simply float off into the ether or twitch my nose to run the vacuum. Life continued and I continued to work toward creating a full, rich life for myself and my family.

As I left Sacred Forest, I recommitted to transferring my writing from paper to laptop for the second wave of fifth chakra. I arrived home safely, empty from my rant and stunned to realize I had left my journal back at Sacred Forest. I could see it in my mind, on the long dining room table behind the chair where our facilitator had sat. The journal contained the second half of my book and intimate details of my journey. *Great. Now I'm naked and exposed. Vulnerable to whoever retrieves my journal and opens it to identify its author.* My stomach queasy, I took a deep, cleansing breath. *All is well. Just let it go.*

What was weird was, leaving my journal behind made my goal attainable. I had only the first part of my journey to transcribe. This was a manageable and necessary task since the first half had been written on loose paper and was scattered about the house: some in the office, stapled together, some in my bedside table drawer, others tucked into books as page markers.

Clearing up the loose pages brought order to my life and

my story. I sat atop the kitchen island and entered the last page at eleven-fifteen the night before the *real* sixth chakra gathering. The holidays over, the pages entered, fifth chakra complete, I slept soundly. I dreamt of the following day's exploration into the unseen and unknown realms of intuition and psychic abilities, and a reunion with my journal. I was caught up and ready to continue my story.

"We write to taste life twice." ~ Anais Nin

PART VII

THIRD EYE CHAKRA

TRANSCEND

In order to see clearly,
you must close your eyes.

RECONNECTING THE CIRCUIT

Sitting on the sunroom floor, I smelled, touched and tasted each item on the plate. Some were clearly not edible. I tasted the gritty texture of earth from the garden soil, and pressed cold steel — a metal screw — against my lips.

I inhaled familiar aromas: deep, intense, tantalizing. Then touched each chocolate chip to my mouth. Their shape changed ever so slightly as they began to warm against my lips. I introduced them to my tongue and took each one slowly inside, tracing their transition from solid to liquid as I rolled them around with my tongue. I swallowed, following the trickle of cocoa down my throat.

At first, the blindfolded expedition proved an exercise in patience, and then, as I surrendered to the slowness, it became a joyful gap in time. No time. Just taste, smell and feel. A cocoon of darkness swaddled me as I licked the escaped droplets of orange from my face.

Alora collected our plates. Music entered the space around me. *Om guruve namaha. Ooooooooom guruve namaha* sang out through the room. The recording of a man's voice ran through my body, intensifying with every repetition of the chant.

The haunting voice fished emotions from me one by one in the darkness. There was no place to put my attention other than the vibration of sound and its effects within. The tone drew a once-buried sorrow to the surface, touching my heart on its way by, releasing tears behind my blindfold. *Om guruve namaha.* Hope swam to the surface, not hope from helplessness but hope from strength. Hope from knowing the human spirit. The sorrow shifted with the hope and my body coursed with the vibrations.

We moved between intuitive postures on our mat — sensing our way into how the body needed to express itself — and chanting. My hands gripped the cool, rubbery surface of the mat, ridged with fine bumps, like a braille sign worn from use. I used it to guide my practice. I emerged in downward dog and paused for a breath. My elbows yielded to movement as my hips swayed side to side, opening, stretching, releasing. My spine arched and twisted, snaking above my mat, awakening my body and releasing any inhibiting movement or thought in the safe cover of darkness.

I was oblivious to anyone else's presence in the room and yet completely aware of their energies. No one was watching. With heightened perception, I reached and opened, expanded and retracted, sensually expressing my body freely in the anonymity provided by the blindfolds. We spent what felt like two or three hours cloaked in the safe space, free of sight, light, time or thought, sensing our way.

"When you're ready, come to sitting. We will continue by smiling up the whole body. Begin with thinking of a happy memory or time. Encourage a smile and allow it to grace your lips. Now draw the smile into the left eye ... then the right. The left ear pulls the smile ... the right ear. Now the brain ... the whole face ... the inside of the mouth, teeth and gums, all smiling, completely happy."

The smile travelled through my body. More spontaneous yoga poses erupted. I felt both empty and full: empty of thought, of form, of physical energy: full of vibration, of breath, of potential. Vast and deep, not bound by space or time, without the border of the room or my body, I sensed limitlessness. I was free to explore a place that required darkness, emptiness, expansiveness: uninhibited and infinite in my connection to that space.

Ajna: command or summoning. The elusive third eye. Sixth sense. Sixth chakra. Beyond wisdom. It's element? Light. Cosmic vision.

"Find stillness in sitting on your mat ... now remove your blindfold." Alora was easy to locate as the blindfold had sharpened my ability to pinpoint her voice. I peeled it from my face. My lashes stuck together. I did the upward under-eye swipe to clear any smudged mascara and prevent the circus clown look.

"We will work with a mudra for sixth chakra." Alora pulled her hands together at her heart. "*Hakini* mudra. We will also use *Bhrumadhya drishti* or eye gaze. Start with the hand gesture. Lightly and evenly press the tips of fingers and thumbs together in front of you with palms apart ... a teepee with your hands."

"Hakini mudra promotes cooperation between the right and left hemispheres of the brain," continued Alora, "memory training, deepened ability to concentrate, and improved and deepened respiration."

I found the mudra comforting, one set of fingers pressing on the others, one side of the body supporting the other. A flow of energy travelled my body as if I'd connected two circuits. My body fed itself in a continuous loop of energy.

"Now for the eye gaze. Close your eyes and fix your gaze between your brows ... expanding backward toward your pineal gland ... deep in the centre of your brain."

My eyes strained.

"Keep the gaze at the centre of the brow," coached Alora. "Not too high or low."

No matter how I adjusted, strain continued.

"Bhrumadhya refers to the point between the brows, the third eye. It is used to stimulate and open that point."

I suspected with further practice, the drishti would become easier as my eyes strengthened.

"Long ago, one either chose spiritual life or family life." Alora's comment poked me right between the eyes. With no family, one might more easily attain enlightenment, but the whole idea of picking one path over another pissed me off. *Why could enlightenment not be attained with a family, through the practices a family afforded?*

The belief survived the generations and lingered for many people, torn between the two. And not just family and spirituality, but work and spirituality or making a life and spirituality. Alora joked that the meditations we learned were set out by monks in caves with no children, jobs, houses or bills to pay, and bodies that could be folded up to look like a scorpion.

"Just do what you can," she reminded us. "Our practices are simply guides."

A merging needed to happen: family and spirituality, life and spirituality — like the circuit connected between the fingers in Hakini mudra.

Still more spontaneous yoga postures followed. Blindfold gone, I continued to move as freely as I had moved in the dark, closing my eyes to return within and devour the deep inner experience, still fresh. I came to rest on my back in savasana. I surrendered to my mat while the entire morning's practice washed over me like waves upon the shore, leaving the sand clean of footprints, residue or debris.

Taking time to come back to my physical self, my breath and the sunroom, I finally encouraged my eyes to open and my body to move into a seated position. My stomach rumbled, bringing me firmly back to my body and the fact that lunch loomed.

"We have one last exercise before lunch. Break off into pairs and find a quiet space in the lodge to explore an intuitive sharing. Sit quietly, face to face, with your partner. Feel into their energy. Wait for a word or thought to arise for the other. When one emerges, share it aloud."

Britt and I partnered and sat on the comfy quilt on top of the bed in the red room. We focused on each other. Then, as per Alora's instructions, we said the first word that came to mind for the other.

"Integrate," said Britt.

I paused to take that in. It struck a chord. I had heard the word used more in recent months than in my entire life. I think few people used it correctly. Britt's insight told me it was time for me to not only understand integration, but to embody it as well.

49

ROUND 1: IT'S IN THE CARDS

"We call on the Spirit of the East," Shaman Karen began, while Alora shook the rattle and helped create sacred space. Sixteen of us sat in circle — more of an oval, defined by the rectangular living room of the lodge. The fire popped in the stone fireplace. The air in the room pushed against me and the temperature began to rise.

"Pick a deck of cards to work with." Karen nodded toward the stack of divination cards on the table."

We each grabbed a deck, no time to contemplate design or author.

"I will guide you through three different dimensions ... levels of intuition ... each one deeper than the previous. Hold your cards in your non dominant hand and think of a question. Nothing too complicated. Something very simple like: 'What is my name?'"

What's the point of that? If I'm going to ask the cards for something, I want answers to the big questions, the tough stuff, not "what is my name?" I'm pretty sure I know that one.

"Am I a mom?" I complied.

I shuffled the deck, stopping where I felt drawn. I turned over the top card to reveal Isis: *you are responsible for many beings, many "children."*

"If the message on the card you pulled prompts a further question, pull another card for more clarity."

I turned over the next card in the deck: *your healing is where it should be, release responsibility for others.* I flipped over another card, intrigued to continue the story: *guiding children.* I paused to contemplate the duality of the two cards. Release responsibility for others, possibly my children, yet use my skills to help children.

In order to help children, I needed to release responsibility for them, release shouldering all of their issues as my own. Once I let go of that weight, maybe I could more freely share my knowledge and their interests, challenges and successes, without exhausting myself. It felt strange to consider giving up responsibility for my kids, but I understood it was the element of blame I needed to release, not the element of care. I jotted down notes in my journal. Another question surfaced.

How do I use my skills to help children? I turned another card. It's message: *go outside and get fresh air.* I pulled again: *boundaries, don't let others take your energy or time.*

I noted the message in my journal. Most of my resentment stemmed from feeling I had no time in a day to do what I enjoyed. I felt guilty taking time for myself while the kids were home. The kids needed time with me and also needed to respect my alone time; when Mom took an hour to herself, that was time to play on their own, in their room or with each other. I struggled to set boundaries with which everyone agreed.

One final card — a vibrant image of a radiant goddess who offered the message: *everything is going to turn out fine, stop worrying.* Worry, something I knew well. I tucked my cards back into their box and set them on the floor next to my chair. I removed my sweater as the room temperature rose.

50

ROUND 2: INTERVIEW WITH AN ENVELOPE

The air felt thick and the room, full, as if it was standing room only. Alora walked around with a basket of letter-sized envelopes. We each picked one. Karen led us into the second dimension. "Focus on the envelope and ask it to reveal its contents or message. Then write down or draw a picture of anything that comes to mind during the process."

I started drawing: a sailboat first, sailing down a gutter overflowing with spring rain. A sailboat made of sticks like we used to make on the farm as kids. The spring runoff would flow from the field, past the horse pastures and yellow bunkhouse, past the hammock strung between three large poplars, and all the way down to the garden.

Next, I drew a ladybug, then balloons and a picnic basket: signs of spring. Finally, I drew a flower. *Is there a stem?* It seemed important to determine if there was a stem. I typically drew the same scene over and over again when drawing with Michael and Khali: grass, a tree, the sun, three birds off in the distance and a flower with a stem and two leaves, one on each side, staggered, one larger than the other. Old habits die hard, but it occurred to me to ask the question of the stem. *No.* There was no stem on that flower.

"Look inside your envelopes," said Karen. A flower sticker. No stem, no leaves, a single flower. *Did I really just do that? Did I really just draw what was inside the envelope?* The most fascinating part was the insight I gained into allowing something to unfold, to lead me down the garden path of inquiry, expanding until I reached the object of my desire.

"Ask if there is a message in this process for you," Karen prompted.

All my images pointed to play outside. It furthered the card inquiry: the outdoors and childhood fun.

Third dimension loomed. "This dimension is called the Mythic. We won't stay in the space long. It is deep and more intense than the others. It requires more energy to hold."

Another basket came around containing envelopes or brown bags for each of us.

"Hold the envelope or bag lightly on your lap. Connect deeper with the contents." My bag felt weightless and I wondered if it contained anything at all.

Sweat pooled at my hairline. My stomach complained about Alora's black bean brownies as the room temperature continued to rise. The air sparked electric: immense energy stirred up by Karen's process.

"It's more important to connect with the message the item in the bag holds for you, than to simply identify the item."

Group inquiry multiplied the energy in a tangible way. I felt claustrophobic and queasy. I wanted to go outside, to have the limitless sky above me and my feet in the grass. I breathed deeply and planted my feet so firmly on the floor, sending my roots into the earth below, that I lifted the front legs of my chair off the hardwood.

Messages came like rapid fire and I tried to write as quickly as they emerged. I sketched when I fell behind. A squirrel: harvest in fall, hibernate and grow in winter, and get busy in spring. A grizzly bear: hibernate, restore, regenerate, grow. Then an eye: open, then closed, hinted at a time to sleep, to recover. I saw a Reiki table with an energetic field above it: store energy.

The rhythms of the seasons and how the animals followed them, called for me to follow them as well. I had harvested much and well in fall, like the squirrel gathering nuts. I needed to sleep, eat, grow, restore and integrate all that my year had cultivated. I opened the brown bag to reveal a walnut.

51

POST AJNA AH HA

Back home, Britt's word, *integrate*, penetrated my mind. During much of fifth chakra and the H1N1 purging, I had bounced between my worlds. One minute I cared for two kids under the age of six, and the next minute, I stood in front of a group of women who were ready to be energized and exhausted by my instruction. Then back to clean up after dinner. Bedtimes came and went, and finally time to do paperwork or a bit of writing. Inspiration would hit and sweep me off into a meditation and chakra clearing, only to be pulled out by a child calling: Mom.

Then I would join a group for a few hours of Reiki-share or a walk, feeling like I could weave the most exquisite web of my life afterward. I would return home to roll up my sleeves and clean up vomit or console someone back to sleep. Feeling whiplash from the two areas of my life, spirituality and family, I surrendered to the possibility the two might never seamlessly merge.

I stood in my pantry, tired from the length of the day, yet charged from the barrage of activities. I stared at the pantry shelves as if I were searching for something. Maybe an answer sat between the rice and the applesauce. A tingling from the base of my spine crept up my back, along the underside of my arms, and continued up my shoulders to the top of my scalp.

I plucked a Halloween-sized container of Smarties and sat down on the plastic footstool at the bottom of the pantry. I poured a red one and a black one into my palm and closed my eyes. Popping them into my mouth, I sucked slowly, squeezing every sensation I could out of those two little confections that I had previously banned from my body. As the hard shell gave way to a softer chocolate centre, I heard what was becoming a familiar voice from within: *Knowing with all that I AM, it doesn't matter what experience I am having, THIS is my experience.* For a moment, I felt no need to juggle or label or separate them into categories. Integration.

I often struggled between ego and self, thinking them separate and, interestingly, one good and one bad. The ego, I labelled bad, thinking altruistic intentions came from the self. Unfortunately, my logic created a rift between the two, an internal struggle between me and myself.

I contemplated integration: all seemingly separate parts forming the whole. It need not require effort or force or figuring or deciphering to merge the various parts of me. It simply required hibernation and restoration. I thought back to the walnut in my brown bag at last weekend's inquiry. Maybe the external work was complete. With the year in yoga nearly concluded, maybe it was time to slip under the blanket of winter, and explore the inner world behind the blindfold.

52

PLEASED TO MEET ME

I headed to Sophie's for Reiki. She greeted me with her usual warmth, asking about my recent yoga gathering. I hopped up onto her treatment table and told her about the events of sixth chakra retreat and my encounter with heightened intuition.

"Well, then," she said. "I have a new focus for our session."

I lay back and slipped between the instrumental music and the neroli oil escaping from her diffuser.

"Close your eyes. I am taking you to meet your inner guide," Sophie continued. "You are standing at the top of a long staircase."

She led me step by step, down the stairs. My toes gripped shaggy carpet as I descended further and deeper into meditation. "At the bottom of the steps you see a large door. See it clearly: its textures and colour. See your hand reaching for the door handle. You open the door and walk through. There is a chair in the room. Sit down."

I looked across the room. It was a large room with wooden plank flooring. A nook with ample windows revealed great green trees and gardens beyond. A comfortable-looking, Victorian-style chair, with a high back and floral fabric, stood in the nook. I sat in the chair.

"Wait. Watch the door for your guide to enter."

I rested in the chair, eyes on the door. My mind crept in to say no one would show.

A man, tall and bald, wearing jeans and a denim shirt, came through the door. He had the most radiant skin and intense blue eyes.

"Nod when you see your guide."

I nodded.

"Embrace your guide and say thank you for coming."

I hugged the tall stranger who felt familiar in my arms, like an old friend. A very dear, old friend.

"Your guide holds a gift for you," Sophie said. "Open your hands to receive it."

I opened my hands.

"Look at it," she continued. "See it clearly. What does it mean to you?"

I looked into my cupped hands to see a soft pink, heart-shaped crystal pendant. I asked my guide what it meant; it seemed to be a present, a welcome gift.

"Thank your guide and leave the room the same way you entered." Sophie guided me back up the stairs, across a bridge and into a meadow where other women waited to receive me. I opened my eyes and brought my awareness back to the music, the scent of neroli and the room. It took time to pull myself from the deep sleep. I wanted to stay in the room with the old friend and the Victorian chair. Sophie poured me a glass of water while I pried myself from the table.

I revisited the process on my own several times over the next few weeks. I made myself comfortable, sitting with a blanket, relaxing music, a candle and, of course, tea. I settled into third eye. I repeated the meditation, step by step, to find the details varied slightly each time. The steps changed from carpeted to granite or slate, or a sparkly stone. The door varied in height and materials, and the room danced in detail. My interior landscape came alive.

Every time, the dear friend met me with deep affection. Every time, more insight unfolded. And, every time, I felt reluctant to leave. The messages were clear, but I couldn't imagine accomplishing what I saw at the time as a great feat — one that would take a lifetime to complete.

I always asked the same question of the bald man in the denim shirt, who I now call Bob, because that name makes me chuckle: "What is my life's purpose?"

At first, he gave me a pen. I liked that, because I liked the thought of being a writer. Of course, I also considered that my clever ego had gotten involved in that pen gift somehow.

The next time I saw him, he gave me an old fountain pen. That made me smile, but I still wasn't convinced my ego wasn't animating the puppet. The third time, a feather quill. *Fine. I get it. I'm supposed to write.* The fact that writing lit me up more than anything else should have been reason enough to accept it as my purpose. As Joseph Campbell said, "follow your bliss," but I was a hard sell.

I returned with the same question. This time, he stepped aside and revealed a floor-to-ceiling, wall-length bookcase that I'd never noticed in the room. Books filled the shelves. Hundreds of them. Bound in old, reddish leather. I rummaged through the house, certain Steve had a couple old books with similar binding. My life purpose must be in their pages.

I returned the following day, no further ahead in my search for the books. I once again asked my question. Bob once again stepped aside and revealed the bookcase. I asked him to show me one so I could see the title or contents. There was no title on the cover. Bob opened the book and flipped through its pages. Blank. Every one of them. He smiled a big smile. I was to fill them.

Hundreds of them?! My excitement over confirming my life purpose of writing turned to exasperation as the weight of those ruddy books crushed me. I hadn't written *a* book, let alone a hundred. I stopped visiting Bob and dove back under the blanket of winter.

The email sharings from the group continued. Mike expressed the duality he found in spirituality and the work-place: livelihood, money. He wrote about the bliss of our gathering, followed by days in the office and corporate life, back to days of yogic practices.

Anna weighed in, having missed ajna weekend, she recommended a book to the group, *The Mind is Mightier than the Sword* by Lama Surya Das.

"It really speaks to the idea of integration," she wrote. Even though she missed the gathering due to illness, she never missed a step. The individuals in the group seemed to function well as a whole, each a part of the living organism of our sangha, our yoga community.

Caroline offered a poem, Mike provided research and commentary on Alora's vegetarian posts, and Gabriella shared a mantra: *Tat Tvam Asi*, "I am that, you are that, that is that, and that's all there is."

Soon came Alora's email detailing the events of seventh chakra, our final gathering. I was stunned by the pace of the year. Sadness seeped in as the end of our journey together neared.

Alora sent a second email requesting referrals. She planned to start the next year in yoga and asked us to share our experiences so that she could include our words in the invitation to the next group. A familiar twinge of uneasiness hit with that particular email. *Is Alora preoccupied with marketing her next service before she'd even wrapped up ours?* In my personal practices of self-discovery, I had forgotten that our year of exploration was also a business: the business of spirituality. I didn't like what was brewing inside me. It was jarring to realize my expansive year of struggle, growth, healing, and vulnerability was a product. Clearly, further integration was required.

Following Alora's email, a covert suggestion came from Nurse Louise; she suggested a group thank you gift for Alora. Of course, everyone agreed, and decided on a compilation of gratitude messages, poems, art and blessings to commemorate her contribution and our year together.

Each agreed to bring their offering to seventh chakra gathering, to insert secretly into the book over the course of our session and present it to Alora at the end. I sat with a cup of tea, inviting my expression of the year to flow onto the page.

Grateful for the year and all that came with it, I still did not connect with her hummingbird ways, and I could only write what I had in me to give. I let go of the need to create a masterpiece of emotion and allowed a simple, humorous poem to pop onto the page.

I spent my remaining days in ajna — restoring, eating, sleeping, enjoying spontaneous yoga, and playing in the snow with the kids. We collected icy flakes on our tongues and scooped mittenfuls of the fluffy white nourishment into our mouths: snow prana. We baked cookies, drank hot chocolate with marshmallows and made generous batches of ribolitta, filling the house with the comforting aroma of Italian stew.

My yoga journey was wrapping up. The year of exploration had matched the rhythms of the seasons: shoots of new growth in early spring, followed by late spring's emotional rains, the heat and intensity of summer's fire, and the cultivating of love and compassion on the fall breeze. Winter provided the darkness and the insulation to dive inward, to float dreamily into inner worlds. Late winter, the imminent time of final chakra, would bring me face-to-face with a new spring.

"The only way of discovering the limits of the possible is to venture a little way past into the impossible."
~ Arthur C. Clarke

PART VIII

CROWN CHAKRA

UNITE

You finally gather all your pieces,
only to realize you, yourself, are a piece of something
greater.

ASHES OF OUR INTENTIONS

A lora and Mike brought the *Awakening the Dreamer* symposium and documentary film to us. "Virtually every natural habitat across the planet is being degraded." Randy Hayes' voice reached me while footage of fires, floods, deforestation and famine flashed across the screen. "How did we get here?" was written across the images. Tears pooled in my eyes. The thought of just what we, humanity, had done to the planet, our home and our global community, broke my heart. It was hard to watch the presentation. I felt helpless to make any impact large enough to matter.

Of all the experiences, all the difficulties the year had shaken loose, this assault on Nature, on Earth and her beings, cut me the deepest. I sat face-to-face with humanity's collective demons. How *did* we get here?

Awakening the Dreamer, Changing the Dream documentary is about the Achuar people of the Amazon, one of the last dream cultures, and how they reached out to modern civilization. They made one request: please change the Western way of thinking from short-term gain to a more viable, sustainable plan for the planet and humanity. Their dreams revealed the need to speak their message to those who could convey its urgency and gravity to the world, motivating and empowering each person to become an agent of change.

The crowning glory to our year had arrived. Seventh chakra, *sahasrara*, Sanskrit for *thousand-fold*, crown chakra, oneness. The itinerary was not at all what I expected. It was not all about me as most inquiries proved up until then. It was clear the *me* part of the journey was opening to the *we* part of the journey, as crown chakra blossomed into oneness.

Many had brought sleeping bags with the aim of sleeping outdoors under the late February full moon. Some placed their bags in the loft, preferring the painted-mandala floor over the snow-covered ground. Anna and I had grabbed the red room. Sleeping on the ground was not on my radar. Even though my back felt better than it had in years, I chose to honour my body and continue the conditions toward healing; and sleeping on the frozen earth was not one of those conditions.

We sat in the living room of the cabin, engrossed in the documentary. I wiped tears from my cheeks. The next images of communities working together, solar energy, wind energy and flourishing forests and crops sprung forth hope from within. It wasn't too late to make a difference.

The fact that I happened to live in a prosperous and safe part of the world positioned me to do something about the degradation of the planet. It positioned me to speak about it and to make changes in my life that aligned with the aim of the symposium: "To bring forth an environmentally sustainable, socially just, and spiritually fulfilling world." All I needed to do was my part, encourage others to do theirs, and in the greatest game of *pass it on*, we could shift the way we related to and lived with the environment, other species, the planet and one another.

The entire symposium was a *bridge the gap* experience, taking participants from an analytical place and shifting them to a holistic place, one of connection, intention and action. The video content, as well as the facilitators, inspired us into action, asking, "What can *you* do?" We brainstormed our responses with each other and recorded our commitments on paper. I committed to get involved with our community garden and to link the garden with our elementary school classes — connecting kids to the earth and their food.

The presentation offered something for everyone: facts, data, a subject that incited emotions and ignited a deep yearning to act. It was powerful. Necessary. I wanted to watch it again and again, to reignite a passion for action and fortify a desire for change *every* day.

"When you say you are going to throw something away, where is away? There's no such thing." Julia Butterfly Hill's words and voice woke me up from the dreamless sleep that was my life, the throw-away world to which I had given little thought. The conveniences of modern life for which I held great gratitude also left me ignorant to the real cost of those conveniences, the cost to the planet, and its inhabitants. I wanted my children to know a healthy world, not spend their lives struggling to heal it or trying to breathe through the ashes.

After the symposium, we pulled on our boots, jackets and gloves, and headed out by car-loads toward Two Pine. Sitting four hours, mired in the world's issues and humanity's responsibility to make a change, proved a lot of information to absorb. As I hiked through the snow, back up the familiar hillside, movement and nature helped my body and mind assimilate all that I had ingested during the symposium and, in large part, our year in yoga. No silent walking meditation occurred on the hike up. No putting on a presence or an appearance. No mind chatter running amok. No feeling out of place or sorts.

Cheerful conversation carried through the barren birch branches as we made our way to the top. Once we hit the steep climb toward the peak, John and Mike raced each other, playfully scrambling up the rocky hill-face.

Overheated from the unusual late February warmth, I removed my jacket near the top of the hill and tied it around my waist. I drank from my water bottle enjoying the cool, fresh water of Sacred Forest. We reached the top and lay down our blankets, Anna and I sharing one. Alora snapped a few photos of us. We sat as bright lights against the subdued hues of late winter.

We stared out over the sun setting on the Canadian Rockies, each of us in meditation, perhaps reflecting on the past year or the year to come, or simply being in that place. With ease and peace, I merged into my surroundings and slipped between the moments in timeless contentment.

I brought my attention toward the centre of the group at the same time as the others, emerging from our place of silence all at once, not guided or planned: a synchronized closure to the meditation. As I turned to the others in acknowledgment, my smile joining with their happy sighs and lightness, one single moth flew out from behind us. I delighted in the unlikeliness of an insect, particularly a winged one, out and about in the still snow-covered hillside. A nod from nature, of a journey well-travelled. Perhaps from the Achuar, Earth and our global community. A recognition of a closing journey and premonition of the one ahead. I had travelled far and yet found myself in familiar surroundings.

The moth symbolized transformation. An insect of night, of moonlit life and dreamtime, the moth emerged from amidst the group, as if to acknowledge our collective waking, that we too held the ability to navigate the darkness and change the dream. We could always find sources of light. Just as the sun set, she flew off to explore the great nectar of night and dreamtime, as the Achuar custom.

Alora brought out a jar containing the ashes of all our intentions — the papers we had written on during our fist gathering, the ones she couldn't light on fire that day. We each took a small amount and found a space on the hilltop to scatter the ashes in a farewell offering. I took a few steps into the community of birches and released my ashes. My intention — *family* — floated amongst the steadfast keepers of the hilltop.

I walked back to Anna's blanket to help pack up. Darkness fell and we needed to make our descent. I leaned down to retrieve my water bottle and noticed something partially buried in the earth directly in front of where I had been sitting.

I dug it from the earth with my fingernails. A bronze trinket of sorts, maybe three inches long, it looked antique. The oval at each end reminded me of a king's sceptre.

The earth had handed me a gift: a graduation present. I stood, uncertain whether I should remove it from the site. Perhaps someone had buried it there as a ritual or blessing of their own. Even if someone had placed it there, maybe it was for me to discover.

I handed it to Mike, thinking with his wealth of knowledge on a variety of subjects, he might identify it.

"Yes." He took it from my hand. "That's a Tibetan dorje."

And he headed off down the trail with it. I assumed he misunderstood my intentions, thought I was giving it to him, and had absconded with it.

"I've been robbed," I told Anna, then promptly tattled to Alora who retrieved it for me.

"Okay that was weird." I turned to Anna, embarrassed. "My reaction ... as if I'd found an ancient treasure and suddenly this anxiety arose at the possibility of someone taking it from me. Maybe I'm holding on a little too tight to what I've learned this year."

Anna softened her eyes as she did when we engaged in personal exchanges. "Well, it was very strange how he took off with it. No word as to whether he intended to return it. Still, good observation on your part."

Back at the lodge, I approached the small altar in the sunroom, complete with a variety of personal items from others in the group. I wanted to place my dorje on the altar, when I noticed a bronze bell with a similar appearance. I placed the dorje next to the bell. Their designs differed but were clearly of the same origin.

54

DINNER AND A SHOW

Hoots and hollers erupted from the kitchen. The feast of Indian food had arrived. We'd worked up huge appetites on our evening hike. The aroma of curry and coriander filled the kitchen. My senses swam in the delicacies, as I savoured the spice, my mouth afire; sparks reached up the back of my throat into my nose and tears responded to douse them. I filled my plate a second time. After a full, gratifying day, leftovers proved scarce.

Satiated, I sank into the leather couch in the living room and contemplated an equally delicious sleep. Sleep, however, was not in the cards. Poi spinning anyone? Once again, we took up the plastic balls with the flashing lights and spun wildly, occasionally bonking ourselves or those too close to us. A lively drum beat shook loose my desire to crawl beneath the sheets. We moved the action out into the night air, under the full moon.

Luca had lit fires inside two free-standing logs he had expertly carved to cradle the blaze. "Swedish log stoves," he called them. Red and yellow crackled from within the stump itself and did not overpower the blue-white moon-light falling around us. The flames danced, striking patterns that rivalled those of the poi balls against the night canvas.

Gabriella joined in the spinning. The music pulsed from inside the sunroom. I stood among the tall trees, captivated by the fully-illumined moon. The lingering snow reflected her soft light, which glistened and sparkled back at the sky like stars gazing in a still pond. The aroma of wood fire escaped on the breeze.

I have no idea how long we spun. Time held no reason to rush us. As the poi spinning wrapped up, we returned to the sunroom to continue our group rhythm with a drum circle. Together, many drums, many hands, one beat. One heartbeat. Well, minus one every once in a while when one of us sneaked out of the circle and up into the loft to add our creative entry into the book of gratitude for Alora. The deep voice of the animal skins combined with tree energy, resonated through the sunroom and the cabin, reverberating my bones as my own heartbeat joined the rhythm.

As Anna re-entered the drum circle, I made eye contact as if to say, "I'm next," and slipped from the hypnotic beat and up the narrow ladder to the loft where the collaboration awaited. A note, poem, drawing, I flipped through the book to see the entries of the others. Each page of the book was a different colour, with organic patterns and details in the corners or running along the sides of the paper, like a tiny elf had stepped in paint and danced across the page. Many generous and unique expressions of gratitude filled the pages, reflecting the generosity and uniqueness of each of its contributors. The words and poems of the group flowed as if sourced from Rumi himself. My contribution, not quite so Rumiesque, reflected my year's journey.

Gratitude book complete, drum circle closed, we headed

off to our respective sleeping quarters to enjoy the dream-time of a full moon. The time came to see who was willing to enjoy the chilly February night. Who would sleep outside?

Anna and I headed to our bed, and stretched out under the down duvet. Anna jumped out of bed. "Let's enjoy the full moon light as we're sleeping." She opened the curtains wide to reveal more than the moon outside our window.

Luca was peeling off his outer wear, and preparing to slip into his sleeping bag, which was laid out next to the fire stumps. Gabriella already occupied the double-wide bag. We assumed it was Alora and Mike cozied up in the other bag opposite the glowing logs.

Anna paused for a moment. "Maybe we shouldn't intrude." She looked at me, still holding the curtain open wide.

"Not so hasty," I replied. "Maybe there will be *two* full moons out tonight."

We laughed as Anna jumped into bed. We continued to enjoy the moonlit show as Luca shed more layers before climbing into his sleeping bag. The vision of Luca in his long johns concluded our last night at Sacred Forest Lodge.

55

BLESSING OR CURSE?

We woke early for morning yoga practice. We stretched and breathed and moved in unison on our mats in the sunroom. A light breakfast of muffins, fruit, and tea followed our practice. Two more guests joined us that day. First, an angelic-looking woman named Lillian. She came to offer a Oneness Blessing to each of us, and she prepared an area in the corner of the sunroom. Lilian sat on a chair while we sat in silence on our mats. When we felt inclined, each one of us approached her and sat or knelt on the floor in front of her, holding an intention. I didn't want to go first, yet I didn't want to wait too long.

I approached Lillian after a few others had gone to her. I knelt for a moment and she placed her hands on my head. She said something but I can't recall what; it was all a blur . I tried to hold a positive intention, wondering exactly what she was doing. Distinctly different from Reiki, no waves or tingling arose. No lights. No voices. Nothing. She removed her hands from either side of my head.

Alora's instructions had included returning to our mats

to lie down to allow the blessing to integrate. Once Lillian had removed her hands from my head and I stood, I felt drawn to go outside. I opened the screen door quietly and stepped out onto the wooden planks. The sun warmed my face, but within minutes of lying on my back on the deck, I wished I had stayed inside. It had looked much warmer than it was, and integrating proved challenging with my body trembling from the cold.

I heard others follow me outside. *Boy, they're in for a surprise once they realize the temperature.* They took up positions around the deck.

I managed to find comfort, and within moments of relaxing my body, he appeared. The Grim Reaper approached and stood at my feet. *What does he want? Am I going to die? Is this a premonition, a warning, a "get-your-things-in-order"? Is it my family?*

A blonde woman placed herself next to him, perhaps to comfort me and alleviate the fear. She looked like a Roman or Greek goddess, dressed in a white sleeveless gown with gold sash around her waist. I used my breath to unclench my jaw, but couldn't breathe the fear away. The only comfort, aside from the gentle woman, is that I *felt* no sense of impending doom. Strangely, as fear paralyzed my mind, my heart seemed to know otherwise. No harm will come. *Then what could it possibly mean?*

Stunned from my vision, I brought my attention back to the cloudless sky, the overhanging tree branches, and the wooden planks beneath my back. I sat up and, for a few moments, looked at the pasture, comforted by life around me; then I silently slipped back inside to return to my mat and the warmth of the sunroom. The others returned inside after me and they all lay silently on their mats. Lillian packed up and left the room. I sat, still quivering. But not from the cold.

I'd assumed after Lillian's blessing, visions of love and light and rainbows lay waiting for me: fluffy kittens showing me my life's purpose. My unexpected *blessing* sat heavy in my gut over the following months. It felt more like a curse.

I tried to make sense of it, to put it into a lighter context and not the darkness that accompanies such a sight. I carried the vision around, revisiting it occasionally over the next year with no more insight than when it had happened. I joked about it to a teacher, describing it like the Monty Python skit: "Who is it darling?"

"It's a Mr. Death, or something, come about the reaping."

The teacher had no further insight than I. "It's a recapitulation of a past life," he said. Whatever that meant.

Only years later, on my birthday, would I stumble across a painting of the Grim Reaper rowing the body of a woman, clad in a white gown with golden sash, out to sea. The painting's description entailed death and rebirth, which, by that time, nearly four years later, I had finally accepted. I laid the old me to rest and allowed myself to emerge anew each day.

And it was okay. It was okay to die to myself. There was no reason to cling to the old or even to the now. My life would never be as it once was, yet, from the outside, not much had changed. I wore the same pony tail, lived in the same house, and shuttled my kids to the same schools. The infrastructure of my life remained intact. My entire inner structure, however, was in a constant state of flux.

56

THE MISSING LINK

I thought I would get to know my boatmates during the year, but I had no idea how deeply I would connect with some of them. Except one. There was one person with whom I felt no connection at all. The quiet, kind and knowledgeable John eluded me. It was as if when John spoke, he spoke a different language or talked about things I didn't understand. I had spent the year in conversation with everyone, except John.

Others seemed completely engaged when John spoke. I'd be like, *was that English? Did he use a complete sentence? Does anyone else think those words don't go together?* I just didn't get him.

I walked into the cabin's kitchen to get a cup of tea. Out of the corner of my eye I saw a man, whom I assumed was John, leaning against the wall near the entrance. I poured my tea and turned around to see a face unlike John's, yet a similar energy signature: grounded, introspective, a wisdom-keeper.

"Hello," I said to the fellow, and returned to the sunroom.

Alora introduced us all to our final facilitator. Leo was a light-hearted, straightforward, witty fellow who had spent over twenty years studying under many of the elders from the Apache and Navajo traditions. His wavy collar-length greying hair and weathered skin, coupled with his energy, gave him the appearance of First Nations descent, though I learned later that Leo was actually Italian.

We sat on the floor in a circle. Leo opened sacred space by calling in the four directions and the ancestors. He then talked for a while about many things. He shared stories of being buried up to his neck in the desert, sealed in a cave for days, and sent on a humorous mission for water, humbled by his elders.

"They handed me a stick and told me to find water. Then they walked up the big hill across from me and sat on top, watching me. I didn't know what I was supposed to do with that stick. I tried to use it as a dowsing rod. That didn't work. Then I tried digging with it, thinking maybe water was just beneath the desert floor. Didn't work either. They sat on top of that big hill chuckling at me until finally one of them waved me up. When I got to the top, I could see a gas station on the other side ... with all the water you could want."

Leo guided us through an exercise in which he had participated many times over the years. "Choose a partner," he said. "Pick someone you don't know very well."

That proved difficult since we had spent the year together. As it turned out, I happened to be sitting next to John.

"Now sit face to face, close, and stare into each other's eyes."

This was no fanciful gazing. Hardcore staring contest stuff. We focused on each other's eyes. No looking away, no laughing or making faces. Relaxed, focused, committed eye contact.

My eyes watered. My blinking became weird as I became hyper aware of it. It suddenly went out of sync, as if my body had forgotten the automatic response: more of a twitch than a blink. I didn't know which of John's eyes to focus on. My mind scattered, taking cover from the discomfort. Then my eyes really started to strain. I purposefully held fast my gaze as strange things began to happen.

John's face changed. Each side revealed its own personality. One side looked younger, the other older. Wrinkles appeared then smoothed away. I held my fierce gaze and relaxed my breath as my eyes acclimated to the practice and resistance withdrew. John's face continued to morph, revealing every emotion it ever wore.

I began to understand the predominant emotions over John's life, as a great empathy set in. As if I could see his life in his face, I saw him. I knew John as I knew myself. In the emotions of his life, the expressions on his face, the masks he wore and the soul he bared, I saw a life lived. Was it mine or his?

"Now, stop gazing and rest your eyes." Leo softly broke through our meditative stare. "That was fifteen minutes."

I felt as if I'd watched the years of John's life for hours. The looks on the faces of the others told me I was not alone in that sentiment. We briefly shared our experiences within the group, each one different.

Alora handed out tiny pieces of paper to each of us. "You're going to write your bucket list. What you desire to experience before you die. Think big. Reach for the stars."

I felt rather empty at that point; winding down, I had to push myself to come up with exciting adventures. I managed a few interesting ones and decided I could add to the list as more developed over time.

"You will pull one of the items from your bucket list and commit to fulfill it within one year."

"What?" I said, reviewing my items. "Shit."

We each took turns placing our bucket list strips into a basket and drawing one out. It was like a lottery draw each time. We all cheered at the selections made as if each person had been awarded a prize: houses, trips, and cars. The basket came to me. I placed my strips inside and hoped to pull something doable. I wanted to commit to the bucket list item as I had the year in yoga, but hiking the Himalayas could prove tough to accomplish with kids in tow.

I closed my eyes, swished the papers around with my hand, holding the intention of something easy, and tentatively pulled out one skinny strip of chance: *Dance the hula on a beach in Hawaii.* I smiled at the words on the paper. *Nice.* The possibility of an island trip. I gathered the remainder of my bucket strips and tucked them into my bag.

Alora and Leo closed the circle, the sacred space, and the year in yoga. We all hugged, then gathered our gear from the sunroom for the last time. As we collected our things, we made the final presentation of the day and the year: our gratitude gift to Alora, the beautiful book our community had created. Many participants took their leave and Alora flipped through the pages. I hugged her again, thanking her for the year.

I walked to the altar to retrieve the dorje. John was there, packing up his bell.

"I've never seen them before today," I said, referring to our objects.

"They are used in Tibetan Buddhist practices. The bell is female and symbolizes wisdom, while the dorje is male and symbolizes compassionate action. Together, they are the path to enlightenment."

John and I walked to the parking area, chatting casually like old friends. We said our good-byes, nearing our cars. John no longer spoke another language, or if he did, I understood it perfectly. What my conditioned mind couldn't do to help me understand John, the practice of presence did.

Compassion was key. Communication was key. But if I couldn't see beyond my own conditioning, how could things change? Eye gazing practice had made me deeply present in the moment: with John *and* me. It didn't mean that I stopped taking action. It meant that I opened my lens of awareness, of possibility, and allowed for a different outcome.

I drove past the main house, down the narrow gravel lane and under the hand-carved wooden sign that read: Sacred Forest Lodge. I had not solved the mystery, could not reveal whodunnit, but felt certain I was on the right track. I turned onto the highway and headed for home.

> *"We shall not cease from exploration. And the end of all our exploring will be to arrive where we started and know the place for the first time."*
>
> — T. S. ELIOT — 1955

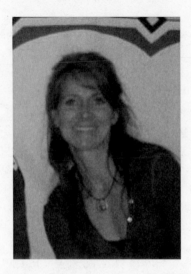

In the teepee at third chakra retreat, pre-fire-walking

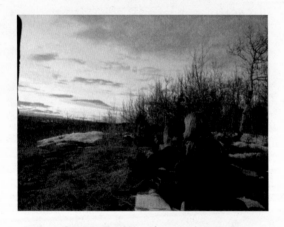

Sunset on Two Pine and our year in yoga

EPILOGUE

~ Dotting the i in Family ~

I slipped the hanger into the purple shirt Grandma had bought Khali for Easter. Purple was Khali's favourite colour and my mom was always on top of those details. Hard to believe a month had passed since Sacred Forest. I missed the cabin and the regular gatherings. I placed the shirt in Khali's closet and headed to the kitchen to retrieve my tea.

On some level, I wanted to have changed more than I had. My incessant thinking was still a concern. I could choose a different thought – often *after* I'd already experienced the habitual thought pattern. But it took consistent effort. I guess that's why it's called practice. It wasn't about changing my nature. It was about *knowing* my nature, and changing my choices.

Awakening the Dreamer propelled me toward sustainable practices and commerce: supporting local producers, investing in clean energy, directing my dollars toward organizations promoting fair trade and women's cooperatives, and taking the time to make choices that benefitted others. Small choices. Made daily. They kept me present and connected to the world and my place within it.

I woke up. I became present. Not all at once. Not all the time. I began to live my life. The life I had spent a lifetime curating. I eventually stopped raising the bar at every turn and simply noticed the insulation of falling snow, the invigoration of a spring breeze, the outstanding wit of Michael, and the pure love of Khali. And I allowed myself to be supported by Steve, who still didn't get it: my love affair with self-discovery and ancient and alternative practices. But I stopped needing him to.

Every breath. Every moment. Full. Not always aware. But I spent more and more time aware than I once did.

I needed the year in yoga to help me unpack years of repressed emotions, decades maybe, unwind them from my spine, and find a more conscious way of living. I needed to know myself and understand my conditioning and behaviour patterns. I needed to know the colour of the lens through which I saw the world.

But at some point, I had to get over myself. I opened up to ways I could be more of service, which were usually right in front of me. Not a grand idea of service, but smaller, immediate acts: the school in need of field trip volunteers or a fruit tray for the Terry Fox run, healthy meals for my family, a non-judgmental ear for a friend, planning a date night for Steve and I, or doing the laundry.

I tugged at the legs of the damp sweat pants. Steve teased me for it, but if I could get an extra half inch out of those pants, Michael might get another month of wear from them. The laundry grounded me. I pulled at the pants with no thought to my back. I didn't have to think about it anymore, because it had been months since I'd known back pain. My mind had moved on to other things. Fear of flare-up had been replaced by the pursuit of happiness.

I turned to tackle the sock pile: what once felt like a mountain. Khali was busy spreading it across the bonus room floor and using the familiar black dress socks as puppets. I smiled as I show her how to fold them together in that balled-up way Mom taught me as a kid.

> **"In every conceivable manner, the family is link to our past, bridge to our future."**
>
> — *Alex Haley*

IN GRATITUDE

I hope you enjoyed *An Accidental Awakening*.

The story didn't end though.

Awakening on Purpose is the 2nd book and the continuation of life after awakening.

To receive the first chapter of *Awakening on Purpose*, visit www.StephanieHrehirchuk.com

If you'd like to explore your own life through the lens of the chakra system, pick up a copy of *Householder Yogini: Chakra-inspired Journaling and Practices for Women who Live at the Intersection of Spirituality and Family*.

And if you enjoyed *An Accidental Awakening*, please leave a review on Amazon or Kobo. It helps others find the book and it helps me to continue writing and publishing inspiring content.

Thank you,

~*Stephanie H.*

ACKNOWLEDGMENTS

To those who walked with me along the journey of awakening.

To Sister Cat, for her constant companionship and ceaseless support.

To the teachers who held the space for lessons and let me discover the wisdom around me and within.

To my husband, for holding fast while my pendulum swung wildly back and forth as I searched my soul and scoured my life lessons for meaning.

To my children, whose tenacity, courage, curiosity, love and humour inspire me every day.

To my parents, who taught me to work hard, make my own meals, stand up for myself and appreciate the value of good neighbours, friends and family.

To my grandparents, who provided a soft place to land when life felt complicated, and memories to last a lifetime.

To you, dear reader, for hearing my story.

I wish you all the love, happiness and joy in the world.
    ~Stephanie H.

ABOUT THE AUTHOR

Stephanie Hrehirchuk is a writer, coach, spiritual seeker and teacher.

Her training includes Tibetan Breathing and Movement Yoga, raw nutrition, spinal reflexology, facial diagnosis, Qigong, Reiki, Ayurveda, plant medicine and sustainability.

Stephanie is the author of *Nourish: Ayurveda-inspired 21-day Detox*, as well as the children's book series: *Anna and the Earth Angel*, *Anna and the Tree Fort*, and *Anna and the Food Forest*. Stephanie has a tree planted for every print copy sold of her Anna series. She donates 10% of profits from *Nourish* to Fuel for School, a Calgary Board of Education initiative that feeds hungry elementary students.

Stephanie was a regular contributor at *Gaia*, with articles published at *Sivana East*, *Finer Minds*, *Guided Synergy*, and *Trifecta Magazine*. She specializes in women's issues. She blogs, coaches and teaches about nutrition, health, yoga, meditation, the chakra system, the world of self-directed publishing, parenting/motherhood and spiritual pursuits.

She still drops the occasional f-bomb. She still hangs out with Anna. She's still writing books. There is never a shortage of tea or dark chocolate.